AF334542

ETHICS ON THE FRONTIERS OF HUMAN EXISTENCE

ETHICS ON THE FRONTIERS OF HUMAN EXISTENCE

Edited by
Paul Badham

An ICUS Book

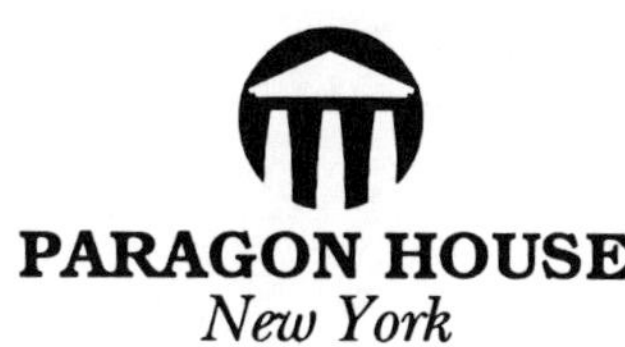

PARAGON HOUSE
New York

Published in the United States by
ICUS
4 West 43rd Street
New York, New York 10116

Distributed by Paragon House Publishers
90 Fifth Avenue
New York, New York 10011

Library of Congress Cataloging-in-Publication Data

Ethics on the frontiers of human existence / edited by Paul Badham
p. 269
"An ICUS book."
Includes index.
ISBN 0-89226-125-0
ISBN 0-89226-126-9 (pbk.)
1. Medical ethics.   2. Human reproductive technology—Moral and ethical
aspects.   I. Badham, Paul.
R724.E821114   1991
174'.2—dc20   90-23696
                                                     CIP

CONTENTS

INTRODUCTION

The purpose of this book is to explore the value of human life, particularly in relation to recent developments in medical research. It is appropriate therefore that the first chapter should set the scene by providing an overview of recent developments in one of the most controversial areas of modern medicine: *Human In-vitro Fertilization and the Present State of Research on Pre-embryonic Material.* In this chapter Simon Fishel, one of the leading practitioners of this science, gives an historical survey of the origins and development of research into human reproduction. He ranges from the speculations of Aristotle 2000 years ago, to the first serious scientific studies which followed the invention of the microscope in the 17th century, and on to the explosion of knowledge which has come with the development of molecular biology following the discovery of DNA in 1953. On the practical front, in-vitro fertilization of mammalian eggs was first attempted at the end of the last century and has been successfully practiced since the 1930's, though the application of this technique to human beings was delayed till 1978.

Dr. Fishel details the procedure followed in in-vitro cases, and gives an account of the early development of the pre-embryo. He presents a forceful case for holding that the pre-embryo should not be regarded as already a person since it lacks almost all the principal characteristics of personhood. Indeed in the first week of life, the human concepti are indistinguishable from other mammalian concepti by even the most experienced embryologist. Concerning the argument from potentiality, Dr. Fishel acknowledges that looking backwards from birth one can indeed trace the origins of each individual to the fertilized ovum, but it is far from clear that it is legitimate to regard the embryo as necessarily a potential person, since even in the normal processes of conception, at least 70 percent of fertilized ova do not go on to become human beings.

Following Dr. Fishel's presentation of the state of in-vitro research, Dr. Robert Winston looks at *The Value of In-vitro Research.* He focuses on the problems of childless couples, and on the joy and fulfillment that the new techniques can bring to some of those who long for a child and for whom this treatment represents their only chance. He also points to the opportunities that this research offers in finding ways to combat that 10 percent of all diseases which we now know to be genetically determined.

The most vocal opposition to in-vitro fertilization today comes from some Christian groups which believe that it is fundamentally wrong. This attitude is explored in detail by Anglican theologian Paul Badham in his chapter, *Christian Belief and the Ethics of In-vitro Fertilization.* He argues that although Christian opposition to research on pre-embryonic material is common, it is hard to see how such opposition can be clearly derived from the sources of Christian revelation. In Biblical terms, life begins at the moment of birth. In Christian tradition, life begins at the moment of "animation." Neither revelatory source justifies opposition to embryonic research. Moreover, reasoning from within the framework of Christian belief makes it hard to justify supposing that "personhood" could be present from the moment of conception since in Christian terms a person is heir to an eternal destiny, and it is difficult to see how such a hope could plausibly be attributed to that 70 percent of fertilized ova which in the course of nature fail to reach even the stage of implantation.

While Dr. Badham's arguments might be persuasive to some Protestant or Anglican theologians to whom Biblical teaching and early Christian tradition are of primary importance, his approach would seem unlikely to cut much ice with Roman Catholic scholars whose revelatory sources also include the living magisterium of the Church today and the supreme authority of Papal pronouncements on matters of faith and morals. Consequently, another chapter is explicitly devoted to *Catholicism and the Value of Human Life.* In this, Michael Coughlan, himself a Catholic philosopher, argues that the claim often made in the context of embryo research that human life is of "priceless value," is hard to reconcile with what the Church has consistently taught in the past concerning capital punishment, or justified warfare, or even the refusal to use "extraordinary means" to prolong human existence. Hence, an "absolutist" stance seems hard to justify without a much more searching inquiry. Dr. Coughlan suggests that the Catholic position, though usually portrayed as based on Natural Law, in fact derives from the Church's understanding of Divine Law. But in his discussion of this he shows that there is very great difficulty in attaching any meaning to the claim that the soul might exist from "the moment of conception." He notes that St. Thomas Aquinas's picture of the gradual development of human personhood is much more in line with modern thought, as well as being the traditional Christian view. He believes that a return to the classic Thomist position, while not requiring the Church to alter its moral stand on the inviolability of the embryo, would certainly alter the seriousness with which in-vitro research was viewed. For in a revived Thomist context, in-vitro research would be banned for the same reasons as contraception is forbidden, rather than as at present being prohibited on the same grounds as murder.

Concern with how to combat infertility must seem something of a luxury to the inhabitants of most countries of the world. Because for them the problem is not lack of fertility, but how to check a population explosion. To this topic we turn in the fifth chapter by Shigemi Kono on *Birth Control and the Value of Human Life*. Dr. Kono vividly illustrates the problems facing the developing countries of Africa, Asia, Latin America and Oceania through the rapid growth of their populations. He shows how improvements in agricultural efficiency are swallowed up by population increase, and how overcrowding, poverty, and squalor diminish the quality of human life. To Dr. Kono the encouragement of family planning is an essential element for promoting the value of human life, but he expresses concern that neither an imposed policy, nor a policy of using abortion as a means of population control should be seen as morally permissible. By contrast with the Third World, Dr. Kono notes that in the rich countries of Europe and North America, total fertility is well below replacement level and the problem of an aging population begins to concern Western governments.

The next chapter is by Christie Davies who explores *How People Argue about Abortion and Capital Punishment in Europe and America and Why*. What he does is to analyze the apparent paradox that supporters of capital punishment tend to oppose abortion, while advocates of liberal abortion laws tend to oppose capital punishment. Both sides defend their positions by claims concerning the value of human life, and yet in almost all countries of the modern West, a shift in public opinion took place in the 1960s against the practice of capital punishment and towards the "liberalizing" of the laws concerning abortion. To explain these developments, Professor Davies propounds his theory of a shift in public thinking from a "moralist" approach where issues are seen in "absolutist" terms of "right" or "wrong," to a "causalist" view whereby actions are considered by reference to their likely consequences. Under the older morality abortion was "wrong" because it offended against an absolutist standard, while capital punishment was "right" because the murderer obtained his just desserts. Under the newer morality, abortion tends to be justified by pragmatic considerations of the likely suffering caused to women by unwanted pregnancy or of resort to illegal and dangerous "back-street" abortionists, while capital punishment is shunned on the pragmatic ground that it does not deter, and hence merely increases the total sum of human misery.

An alternative method of procedure is that recommended by Nicholas Kittrie in his chapter *"Wanted" and "Unwanted" Life: The Impact of New Science on Ethics, Law and Public Policy*. What Professor Kittrie argues is that the contemporary debates reveal a clash between those who can be described simply as "pro-life" and those who can be described as "pro-quality of life." Those who take an "absolutist" stance against birth control, in-vitro fertilization and euthanasia see the presence of life to be protected from the earliest moment of conception to the last moment at which life can by any means be preserved in the human body. By contrast, those who place their emphasis on the quality of life will not see genuinely personal life as present unless and until distinctively valued qualities come into being, nor will they be concerned to preserve bare physical existence if all that is of value to that individual has ceased to be possible.

Dr. Kittrie notes that in the past, discussion has focused on unwanted life in the context of abortion and euthanasia, whereas in the present debate the discussion revolves around wanted life. Those who desire in-vitro fertilization, donor insemination or surrogate mothering desperately want to bring life into the world, and those who resort to heroic measures of organ transplantation or exhaustive and expensive treatment equally desperately wish to keep life in being. It is odd in many ways that the abortionist and the in-vitro fertilizer should be bracketed together, for their whole *raison d'être* is utterly different.

Another problem area is discussed by Helga Kuhse and Peter Singer in a chapter entitled, *Hard Choices: Ethical Questions Raised by the Birth of Handicapped Infants*. They spell out just how severe, limiting and agonizing are the sufferings which can be endured by extremely premature, or seriously handicapped infants, and they call in question the pressures placed on doctors to preserve life at almost any cost, in terms of suffering for the child and its relatives, and in terms of expertise and resources to the community. They note that a painful decision often has to be made in the best interest of the patient to withhold pointless treatment and allow the suffering child to die. However, she raises the question of whether this stance is really in the best interest of the patient. "Letting die" often means a slow and painful death. In circumstances where death is inescapable, would it not be morally preferable to help the child die painlessly and quickly?

The Appropriate Medical Care of the Terminally Ill is taken further in the next chapter by Jan Kryspin and Heather Phillips. They argue that our society must learn anew how to come to terms with death. The transience of life is fundamental to the human condition and should not be regarded as something to be fought at all costs. They commend the hospice movement with its goals of pain control and the provision of the optimum quality of life for the dying patient. They also urge the importance of the personal dimension in the doctor's care for the individual as a unique person, and the need to move away from a technology-dominated understanding of the role of medicine.

A different approach to this question is provided by Patrick Nowell Smith who argues for *The Right to Die*. His view is that the universally acknowledged "right to life" carries with it the right to choose to die, for it is basic to all "rights" that they can be exercised or not at the option of the right-holder. Yet, almost all societies place an enormous obstacle in the way of our right-to-die, by refusing to permit anyone to assist us, even though the cooperation of others is usually necessary for the preferred forms of self-deliverance. Dr. Nowell Smith challenges the classic distinction between passive euthanasia (letting die) and active euthanasia (killing) claiming that this distinction is both illogical and immoral. Once it is apparent that a person's death is inevitable, it should be permissible for him to request, and be given, assistance to die swiftly and painlessly. He notes that this is in practice in the Netherlands, and that opinion polls show wide support for comparable developments in other countries.

Finally, Peter van den Dungen turns to the issue of war in the concluding chapter on *Justified Warfare and the Relative Value of Human Life*. He draws attention to the paradox that many moralists who speak of the absolute value of human life in the contexts of abortion and euthanasia adopt a very different understanding of the value of human life in the context of justified warfare. Moreover, even those who do maintain a strong theoretical opposition to warfare tend to find it almost impossible to maintain their position when the fundamental values of their society are threatened. Dr. van den Dungen illustrates these points by a wealth of historical examples, and argues that the persistence of the idea of justified warfare shows that, in practice, societies and individuals recognize many values as being of greater significance to them than their own personal safety. It is important that these values be recognized not only in discussion of the legitimacy of defense, but also when we seek to explore the ethical dilemmas which arise at the beginning and end of life.

ONE

HUMAN IN-VITRO FERTILIZATION

AND THE PRESENT STATE OF RESEARCH ON PRE-EMBRYONIC MATERIAL

Simon Fishel

Abstract

Should mankind delve into the mechanism of human conception? Should we be interested in how a sperm fertilizes an egg and how the conceptus develops into the embryo, how a conceptus may become an abnormal fetus, or how the normal fetus may be aborted? Should we even ask the questions? What about the infertile couple? Should we ask why they are unable to conceive and how we can help them?

Not all these questions are new to our generation; the plight of the infertile has been heard throughout the ages and was recorded in biblical times. But our generation has witnessed a surge in technical feats; we are the bearers of new knowledge. Facts are emerging on how conception occurs and why it goes wrong. With such information it is now possible for mankind to intervene in its own reproduction. Simple in-vitro fertilization techniques can circumvent many of the initial problems of conception where simpler techniques failed, conceptuses can be cryopreserved, gametes and conceptuses can be donated, and research possibilities exist to discover and perhaps correct disorders in the human conceptus.

No previous generation has had to ask the questions about its own procreation that we now face. How shall we meet this challenge? Only from a position of knowledge! This paper briefly examines the interest in procreation by men and women throughout the ages, leading to the birth of the first child conceived extracorporeally. It examines the arguments pertaining to the nature of the human conceptus from a scientific viewpoint and why many people feel uneasy about the status of the human conceptus. The current practice of "high-technology pregnancies" for the alleviation of infertility is discussed. Finally, the current and future areas of research are also examined, with speculations on the possible advances for the future and with the discounting of some of the more fanciful and sensational but improbable claims, such as ectogenesis and cloning.

Introduction

In recent years much has been written on human in-vitro fertilization and its science, medicine, social problems and ethical issues. Discussions on the ethics of in-vitro fertilization have not resulted in a single authoritative approach, which is not surprising. The Jewish ethic is somewhat different from the Christian ethic; what is deemed ethical by the British Medical Association, the Royal College of Obstetricians and Gynecologists, and the Medical Research Council of Great Britain has been considered unethical by the Royal College of General Practitioners; and the decisions and the dissensions apparent during the investigations of the Committee of Enquiry into Human Fertility and Embryology ("Warnock Report") by members of the Committee highlight the different ethical approaches taken by different groups and individuals.[1]

One of the main problems in sifting through the opinions on the ethics of in-vitro fertilization is the apparent lack of knowledge on the actual processes involved, the research being carried out and the status of a human conceptus. The latter causes the most concern because there is no clear authority on what a human "conceptus" actually is. There are essentially three opinions: (a) the conceptus is a human person (*per se* or with potential); (b) the conceptus is a potential human person; or (c) the conceptus is a few undifferentiated cells with the genetic constitution of *Homo sapiens*. The last is, *prima facie*, a starting point but, as I shall endeavor to explore, is not axiomatic.

Another fundamental point of concern is the moment of fertilization, that is, the penetration of human egg by a single sperm. For many, fertilization is also the moment of conception—that point in time and development when a person is conceived and the soul comes into existence. But recent scientific knowledge suggests that the moment of fertilization ought not to be considered the moment of conception, and even conception may not be considered the formation of a new human person. Some express the belief that penetration of the egg by a spermatozoon is, in itself, an occurrence that should occur inside the body and solely after sexual intercourse.

Until there is agreement on the procedures used by "assisted" human reproduction and a consensus on the nature of the conceptus, it will remain extremely difficult to tackle the problems of pre-embryonic research. I wish to describe the clinical and scientific processes involved in human in-vitro fertilization from a historical perspective that includes today's current knowledge and to associate our understanding with the ethical and social issues. It will then be possible to examine the future areas of research.

Historical Perspective

"P'ru ur'vu" ("Be fruitful and multiply," Gen. 1:28, 9:7)—a divine directive; man was formed "in the image of God" (Gen. 1:27)—a statement describing man's share in God's creation, a being with consciousness and free will; "Give me children or else I die!" (Rachel; Gen. 30:1)—an age-old cry of despair.

From the earliest recorded times, infertility has been a human problem causing great concern, but the lack of fundamental knowledge prohibited understanding. Aristotle was one of the first to question the origins of conception: whether the embryo is preformed and merely unfolds and develops or whether it is a formless mass gradually differentiating into a complex structure, the complete individual. Aristotle favored the latter, that is, "epigenesis"—but the problem remained unsolved for 2000 years.

The development of the microscope was of major importance in the understanding of reproduction. Anton van Leeuwenhoek constructed "home-made" microscopes, observed many specimens and made the first drawings of spermatozoa from different species. After this revelation, in the 17th century, two diverse opinions were mooted: (a) that the sperm contained the individual, the homunculus curled up inside the head of the sperm; or (b) that the egg contained the individual. These views represented the *preformation hypothesis.*

By the end of the 17th century, only two men were recorded as believing in epigenesis, Aristotle and William Harvey. Harvey's famous statement, "Ex ovo omnia" (Everything from the egg), from his work *Exercitationes de generatione animalium,* demonstrated his belief that it was the egg that was a formless mass from which the embryo developed into the individual. This was given considerable support by Charles Bonnet, who in 1745 convincingly demonstrated that unfertilized nonmammalian eggs had the occasional potential to develop into normal individuals—that is, parthenogenesis (see below). Later work on chicken eggs by Caspar Friederich Wolff in the latter half of the 18th century demonstrated the development of the egg from its early cell divisions to the multicellular, complex, embryonic structure. This progressive differentiation was further advanced in 1822 by Karl Ernst von Baer in his work *Developmental History of Animals.* This new knowledge revealed the facts of early embryology for many species and dealt the final blow to the preformation hypothesis.

It was during this period that arguments abounded about the cell. There were two fundamental theories in the 19th century: cell theory and spontaneous generation. Matthias Schleiden believed that the cell was the essential unit of the living organism, and Theodor Schwann's research led him to the conclusion that mammalian eggs were essentially cells. But Schleiden and Schwann believed that the formation of cells occurred by a spontaneous chemical process. In the middle of the 19th century, Ramak and Rudolph von Kolliker demonstrated that the change from egg to embryo occurs by a process of cell division. Further, Rudolf

Virchow demonstrated that one cell could be generated only from a pre-existing cell—thus, his famous quote about the cell: "the last link in the great chain of subordinated formations that form tissues, organs, systems and the individual." Consequently, the Schleiden-Schwann theory of cell formation was denounced. One of the major discoveries in the mid-19th century was that the egg would not develop without a sperm's being present. But even during this period, it was still believed that the sperm was simply a triggering mechanism that switches on the developmental process inherent in the egg. As we shall see later, this belief has, to a certain extent, some scientific validity.

Toward the end of the 19th century, Hertwig and Fol demonstrated the presence of two nuclei (the male and female pronuclei) in the cytoplasm of the fertilized egg. In biological terms this was a crucial discovery, for it was for the first time evidence that the unit binding successive generations was shifted from the cell to its nucleus. Subsequently, major research programs were initiated to search for substances which could be defined chemically and which were passed from sperm to egg. Eventually, threadlike structures were observed in the cell during its period of cell division. Wilhelm von Waldeger-Hartz named these structures "chromosomes."

Also toward the end of the 19th century, Gregor Mendel, a Bohemian monk, made what was later to be a major impact on biology with his law of segregation (stating that, as germ cells form, the two factors for each characteristic separate from each other and end up in a daughter egg or germ cell) and the law of independent assortment (stating that the maternal and paternal factors which separate, do so independently from those of the other germ cell). Considerable research on the chromosomes then resulted in the postulate that actual physical units were located at definite positions along the chromosomes; these units were eventually named "genes."

After World War II came the dawn of molecular biology. Further developments in the sciences of biochemistry and molecular biology had an enormous impact on science and society, not least in the present day, with their relationship to embryology. In 1953, the famous work of James Watson and Francis Crick elucidated the molecular structure of DNA, and researchers eventually were able to demonstrate how genetic coding produces the necessary instructions for the synthesis of all other molecules within the cell. Since the 1960s, this work has enabled scientists to understand the basic principles of how a species can reproduce its own kind; continued research has developed into the now notorious field of genetic engineering. This area will enable scientists and doctors to investigate specific hereditary characteristics that are evolved or suppressed in future generations, and perhaps in the eradication of disease and abnormality it will have a major impact on the future of human embryology. So much for the scientific developments leading to the understanding of fertilization, embryology and the fine structure of the cell.

For more than a century, clinicians have been trying to help infertile couples. It was not until the late 18th and early 19th centuries that specific physical problems were associated with infertility. During this period it was recognized that the Fallopian tubes may be a cause of sterility; and in 1849 a British gynecologist, Tyler Smith, attempted to catheterize the Fallopian tube by the passage of a whalebone fiber through a silver catheter.[2] This method was never officially adopted.

Many surgical approaches were attempted from the end of the 19th century on, including the grafting of ovarian tissue into the oviduct or ovarian grafts to restore ovarian function in women undergoing premature menopause; also, the method known as the Estes operation[3] of grafting the ovary onto the uterus has been used over the last 60 years. Since the end of the 19th century many workers, mainly in Europe, developed techniques for investigating the pelvis and the reproductive organs without any major operation. This eventually led to the ability to visualize the ovary directly (and the follicles growing within the ovary) by means of a laparoscope. It was only a matter of time before human eggs were to be recovered.

It must not be overlooked that another major area that needed to be developed over the centuries was an understanding of the function of hormones (endocrinology) specifically related to infertility. Enormous developments have been made over the last 100 years and particularly in the last 70 years, where the interrelationships among the hypothalamus, pituitary and ovary have enabled scientists and doctors to understand in great detail the reproductive cycle and the human menstrual cycle. One of the great advances in fertility was the development of drugs that enabled women to ovulate under controlled conditions. As will be explained below, for women who require in-vitro fertilization but were ovulating normally, the use of these drugs for this purpose revolutionized the success of the treatment but facilitated the collection of conceptuses for research, thus creating many of the ethical problems.

The first attempts at in-vitro fertilization were performed by the Viennese embryologist S. Schenck in 1878.[4] Schenck worked with rabbit and guinea pig eggs; but although he did not convincingly demonstrate fertilization and further development in vitro, by the end of the 19th century many researchers had investigated this problem in different species. The first publication of successful in-vitro fertilization of mammalian eggs with subsequent birth came in the 1930s with G. Pincus and E. Enzmann.[5] Again, controversy arose and some believed that fertilization had occurred in vivo (valid proof: observation of the pronuclei not made). However, Pincus and Enzman did the early pioneering work and laid the foundation with fundamental observations on the stages associated with fertilization of mammalian eggs. Interestingly, all the morphological events associated with fertilization also were observed for the parthenogenetically activated egg (spontaneous division of the oocyte into the early cleavage stages without fertilization; see below).

Further studies in the United States with N. Menkin and J. Rock in 1946 and 1948[6] led to the first published photographs of two- and three-cell human conceptuses in the *American Journal of Obstetrics and Gynecology*. It was claimed that these had been successfully fertilized in vitro. A few others in America continued this work, and it is interesting to note that infertile women also were becoming interested; it is recorded that infertile women were requesting in-vitro fertilization as a treatment of their sterility caused by absent or blocked Fallopian tubes. It was recognized in 1955 by L.B. Shettles that the treatment of infertility was possible by in-vitro fertilization[7] and this opinion was shared by a few others. With foresight J. Rock explained that Shettles, using a laparoscope, would eventually be able to extract an egg from the ovary, fertilize it in vitro and return the conceptus to the uterus: "Thus, he [Shettles] will impregnate the women in spite of the fact that she has not tubes." It was 23 years before this vision became a reality. In the 1950s in America the climate toward human in-vitro fertilization was hostile, and with the retirement of Rock in 1956 came a decline in interest.

During the 1950s and 1960s major advances were being made in reproductive biology. Significant discoveries enabled scientists to grasp in detail the mechanisms associated with fertilization and the early development of the conceptus. It was only a matter of time before an interest in human gametes would be stirred once again. By the time Edwards and Steptoe started their work in the 1960s, major advances had been made in the fields of laparoscopy, infertility and endocrinology, and, most significantly, in the fundamental processes delineating the events associated with mammalian fertilization and development in vitro. Stringent application of this knowledge by Robert Edwards and Patrick Steptoe in 1978 led to the birth of the first human after conception in vitro. Around the world today more than 4,000 babies have been born by the process of in-vitro fertilization. Had the social climate been different in America during those very early pioneering days, we could be discussing the second generation of children conceived by in-vitro fertilization!

Conception and Misconception

In global terms the problem of infertility is huge; in terms of family and social relationships it can be devastating. It is not in the gambit of this paper to discuss infertility *per se*, but I wish to present briefly the size of the problem. In a recent survey in the United States, it was estimated that the incidence of subfertility in women had risen in the last decade from 10 to 14 percent. About seven million couples are unable to plan a family. This figure represents about three times the number of annual deaths. Of these seven million, approximately 43 percent are sterile, 40 percent are substerile, and 17 percent will achieve spontaneous conception after a long interval, usually of more than six years. In the case of tubal infertility (absent, blocked or diseased Fallopian tubes), it is estimated that 100,000 women suffer from this condition in Great Britain.

Apart from tubal disease, there are numerous other causes of infertility, which are briefly listed in Table 1-1. In-vitro fertilization can be effective in all the conditions listed in Table 1-1. In the main, one of the largest groups of infertile patients is that of those who fail to ovulate. They can be treated by the use of fertility drugs with no recourse to in-vitro fertilization. Since in-vitro fertilization has become more successful and professionals and laymen are more aware of the advances and successes of in-vitro fertilization, many unusual causes of infertility (such as premature menopause and absence of the vasa deferentia) are being successfully treated. In-vitro fertilization is not a technique limited to a very few. In-vitro fertilization is not a mystical technique dogged by complicated procedures and inexplicable methods. Today, it is becoming a relatively simple procedure.

TABLE 1-1

Indications for In-vitro Fertilization

Absent or damaged Fallopian tubes

Semen problems
    oligospermia
    asthenospermia
    teratospermia
    immunological

Blocked or absent vasa deferentia

Endometriosis

Female antisperm antibodies

Unexplained infertility

Premature menopause

Absence of ovaries

Briefly, to achieve in-vitro fertilization, eggs need to be collected during the period when they are mature and receptive for fertilization. They must be collected from the follicle (which is situated in the ovary) a few hours before ovulation as few can be recovered once ovulation has occurred. Two main methods are used to recover the eggs:

1. Direct visualization of the follicle with a laparoscope—hence a minor operation but with general anesthesia.

2. The more recent and very successful procedure of visualizing the follicles by ultrasound scanning and without an operation aspiration of the follicles under local anesthesia.

The eggs must then be washed and maintained for a few hours in a viable culture fluid, which is generally a simple salt solution supplemented with the woman's serum. Semen is obtained by masturbation and washed with a culture fluid parallel to that used to incubate the eggs. A careful assessment is made of the numbers of sperm needed to inseminate the eggs. Generally, the gametes are mixed in the culture fluid within approximately six hours after the recovery of the eggs. They are maintained in an incubator at body temperature for another 20 hours, when they are then removed. At this stage, the eggs are closely examined to see whether fertilization has occurred. The egg is surrounded by thousands of follicle cells (cumulus cells, Figure 1.1) and any selection of sperm will probably occur by the natural processes of the swimming of sperm through these cells, attachment to the outer investment of the egg, and a single one eventually penetrating into the egg. Once apparently normal fertilization has been observed, the fertilized egg is placed in a fresh culture medium and maintained in the controlled environment for another 24 hours. At this time, the egg generally has undergone one or two cleavage divisions, to the two-, three- or four-cell conceptus (Figure 1.2a), at which time it is placed in a catheter and returned via the cervix to the womb. During the first five or so days, the total size (mass) of the conceptus is the same as that of the egg; that is, the increase in cell numbers is brought about by the egg cytoplasm's splitting. Hence, each subsequent cell is smaller than its parent one. At this stage the size of the egg or the conceptus is more than five times smaller than the period at the end of this sentence. The success of the whole procedure depends not only on the expertise of the practitioners but also on stringent adherence to protocol; as Francis Bacon said, "Nature to be commanded must be obeyed."[8]

The process described above has been tried and tested over many decades with hundreds of thousands of mammalian eggs of different species, with no shred of evidence to suggest an

10

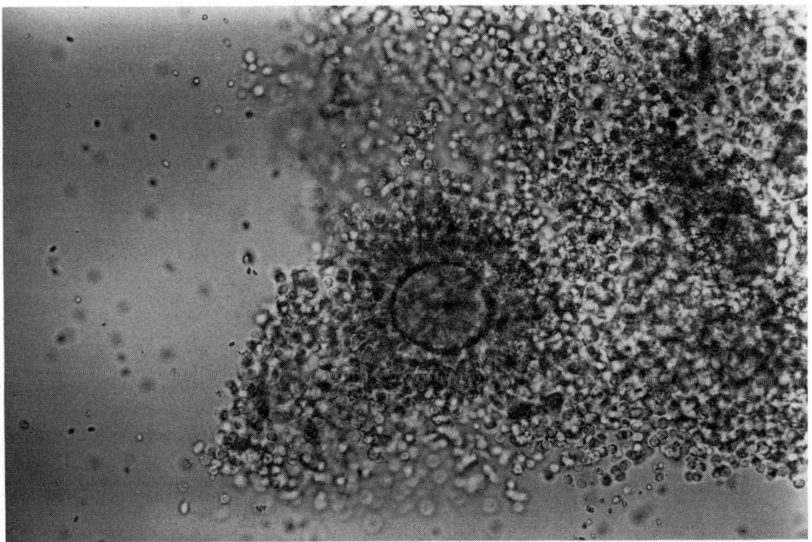

Figure 1.1

increased incidence of abnormality at birth due to fertilization in vitro. The process also has a certain number of safeguards that may lead to fewer abnormalities occurring after in-vitro fertilization than occur after conception in vivo. For example, oocytes are recovered under controlled conditions and insemination usually occurs at an optimal time during the maturation of the egg. In the human female, fertilization in vivo may take place during unfavorable conditions. Unlike many mammalian species, human beings do not necessarily have intercourse during a receptive period around the time of ovulation. Therefore, spermatozoa may be present for long periods of time in the reproductive tract before ovulation, or an egg may have been ovulated a long time before it comes into contact with spermatozoa in the Fallopian tube. The human species is noted for its extremely high incidence of abnormalities, resulting in spontaneous abortion or occurring at birth, and 70 percent of the conceptuses degenerate during or shortly after implantation.[9]

It is generally believed that the moment when the sperm penetrates the egg is the moment of conception. However, conception *per se* is probably not the particular event. As mentioned

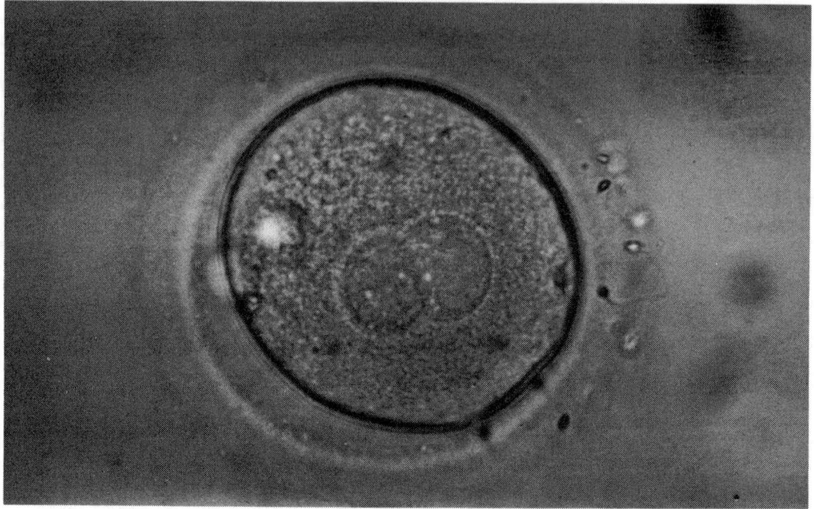

Figure 1.2a

earlier, it is necessary to check the consequences of fertilization some 20 hours after insemination. It is at this stage that the pronuclei are observed, as first described by Hertwig and Fol at the end of the 19th century (see above). One pronucleus (generally the larger) contains the chromosomes, the packaging of inherited information from the father, while the other pronucleus contains the genetic information passed on from the mother. At this stage, perhaps 20 hours after the sperm had penetrated the egg, there is still no "mixing" of the genetic information, and no distinct genetic identity has yet emerged. (See Figure 1.2b) Within the next few hours, the membranes surrounding the pronuclei will break down, after which fusion of the genetic material, syngamy, actually occurs—perhaps this is the moment of conception?

This "normal" sequence of events may still hide serious anomalies which have arisen in the genes or chromosomes and which could affect the development of the conceptus. These insidious and often deleterious genetic or chromosomal defects likely will go undetected. More gross errors also can arise during this period. For example, more than one sperm may enter the egg, resulting in the formation of three or more pronuclei; (See Figure

1.3) and even this abnormal situation does not have a single scenario. Further events will determine the future development of the conceptus, and in theory these may be as follows:

1. One of the male pronuclei may be extruded or not take part in syngamy; this leads to the generation of normal syngamy between a male and a female pronucleus, which results in a full diploid (46 chromosomes) complement in the conceptus.
2. The female pronucleus may be extruded or fail to take its place in the fusion of the chromosomes, resulting in the so-called androgenome, which can be of XX or XY origin with 46 chromosomes—this clearly has no potential for development to a term baby, but it does have some potential for development, as will be described below.
3. All three pronuclei could fuse and result in the formation of a conceptus containing 69 chromosomes, which has potential for development with serious consequences.

Each of these situations may arise after conception in vitro because the final scenario for each (as described below) actually occurs in utero. There is also the possibility that abnormalities that arise during fertilization, gross or subtle, could be corrected or changed during the early developmental period of the conceptus and future embryo. For example, it has been postulated[10] that the differences observed in Down's Syndrome babies, from the high grade to the low grade, may be due to the original anomaly at fertilization that is gradually being corrected by the conceptus during its early development and results in a mosaic with various proportions of defective and normal cells. The high-grade Down's infant will then be a mosaic containing a high percentage of normal cells.

The above examples demonstrate that the moment the sperm enters the egg, a unique, unchangeable, and irretrievable conception does not occur. Life does not arise spontaneously, and many assert that it is a continuum from the life existing in the sperm and the egg. The moment of sperm penetration is an important event in the process of species procreation, but there are further significant events to follow.

In the normal series of events from fertilization, the conceptus will undergo cleavage for about seven days. The word "cleavage"

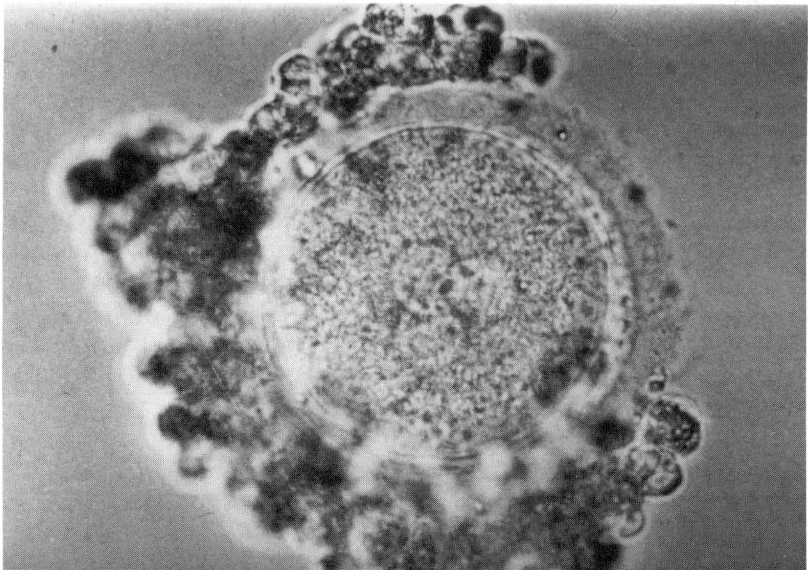

Figure 1.2b

is used rather than "growth" because this stage of development is a unique form of growth. Each egg is surrounded by an outer membrane, called the *zona pellucida*. (See Figure 1.2c) This membrane is cellular and of fixed size. It helps keep the cells of the conceptus intact; during the first three or four days after fertilization each cell of the conceptus is an individual unit and not connected to the next cell; thus, without the outer membrane these cells would fall apart. For the construction of the embryo each cell must have its correct orientation to receive further instruction on its eventual function (the concept of epigenesis)— at this stage the function of each is undetermined. By four days there may be 50 cells, but the actual mass, or size, of the conceptus is the same as that of the unfertilized egg, there simply having been an increase in cell number accompanied by a reduction in cell size.

This period of cleavage is also unique in another way. The individual cells up to the four-cell conceptus are *totipotent*—that is, each cell has the unique capability of forming a complete

14

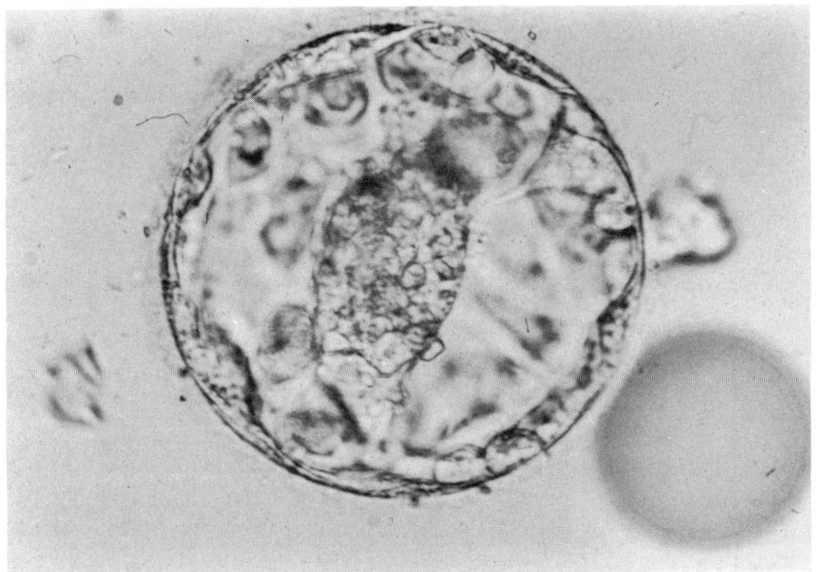

Figure 1.2c

individual. Each cell, like every other cell in the body, has identical information, but at this early stage (unlike those in different tissues of the body, which have become highly differentiated) differentiation has not taken place. It is feasible (and it has been demonstrated in animals) to take a four-cell conceptus, remove the outer zona pellucida, put each individual cell into an "empty" zona pellucida, and let each continue to cleave and develop normally from pregnancy to term to end up with identical quadruplets. This characteristic of each — totipotency — eventually ceases as the cells mature. At about the 16-cell stage, a transformation occurs whereby each cell starts to fuse with another and totipotency is lost. Owing to simple topological positioning inside the conceptus, some cells will be forced into the inside while others remain on the outside. This perhaps arbitrary occurrence is a significant event. By the fifth day there is a ball of cells on the inside with a covering mass of cells on the outside. This particular stage is called the blastocyst and it is still surrounded by the outer membrane. (See Figure 1.4) By the sixth day this blastocyst will

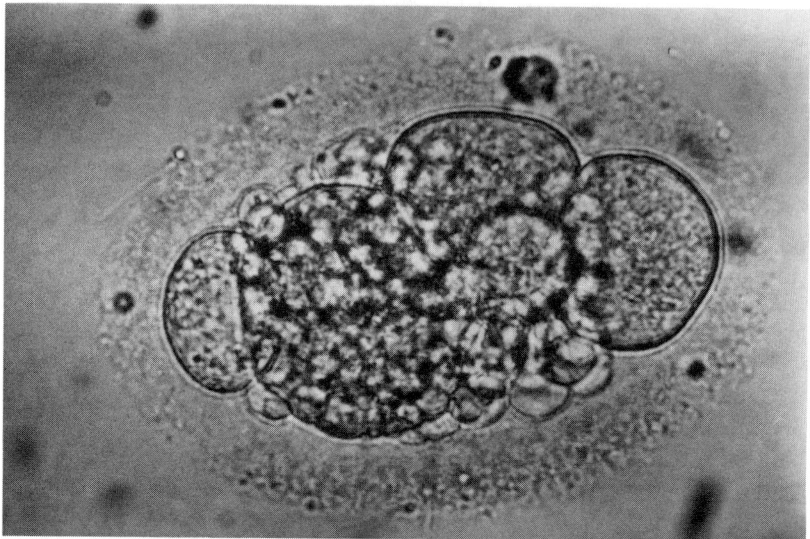

Figure 1.3

eventually "hatch" out of the zona pellucida, attach itself to the lining of the womb, and eventually burrow through; this is the process of implantation that occurs between the seventh and ninth days. Implantation itself is another unique event in the establishment of the future developing fetus.

The small ball of cells on the inside of the conceptus is, at this particular stage, very different from the outer layer of cells. The outer layer of cells is destined to become the placental tissue. These cells have no future whatsoever in the actual makeup of the fetus or baby *per se*, which is made up solely from the mass of cells in the center (which will eventually differentiate and become the embryo). Even during this stage, a single unique fetus is not the only possible outcome: The embryo may split and form an identical twin; and although the genetic constitution of the two would be identical, the outcome of their development may be different. This begs the question of "ensoulment" of the identical twin: At conception or eight or more days later when the conceptus splits?

16

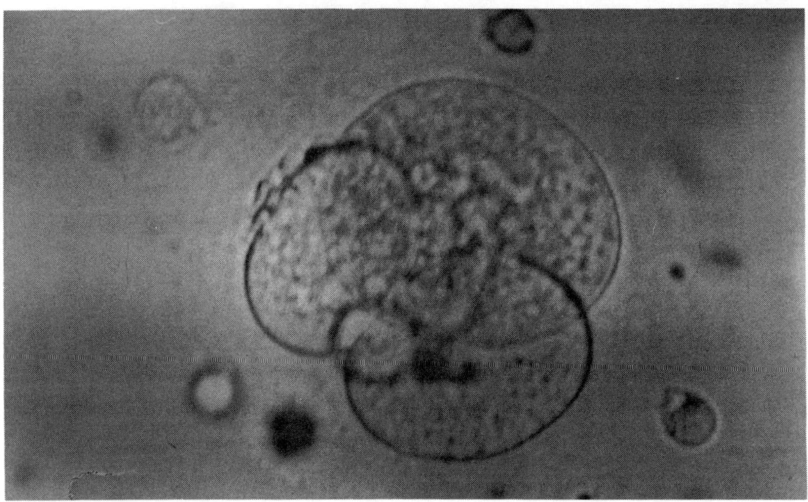

Figure 1.4

I started this section by describing the normal events of fertilization and then an abnormal event (three pronuclei), proceeding to the normal events of cleavage. But even if we consider fertilization and cleavage as a single process, there are other unusual situations that can arise. For example, although a sperm may never penetrate, or even be in contact with the egg, yet the egg may divide and undergo cleavage to quite an advanced stage. This type of cleavage also has more than one scenario. For example, the egg, which initially contains half the complement of chromosomes, may develop as such or may "hold back" one cleavage division and double up its number of chromosomes (that is, the nucleus replicates but not the cell itself), thus producing a conceptus with the diploids complement of chromosomes but without sperm involvement! This is called the "gynogenome," the nearest thing to a spontaneous clone of the mother (although not exactly, as each gamete is a unique entity; see above). The activation of the egg without sperm is termed "parthenogenetic," and parthenogenesis can occur spontaneously in many mammalian species; there is now direct evidence to show that it occurs in humans.

For some reasons, many not understood, the conceptus may cleave normally for one, two, three, or four days and then cease to cleave. Then some conceptuses may degenerate and some may linger on, while others maintain a normal appearance for a number of days but do not divide. This phenomenon, called "cleavage arrest," has been documented for a number of mammalian species, including humans.

If there is one point that practitioners and researchers in the field of in-vitro fertilization agree upon, it is that there is no means of assessing the viability of a conceptus (unlike a person!). The shape and appearance of a conceptus is no guide to its viability. Irregularity of the blastomeres, unusual fragments, and other "ugly" manifestations of a conceptus may occur in those which give rise to perfectly healthy babies (see Figure 1.5), whereas while many perfectly healthy-looking conceptuses (for example, polyploids or parthenotes) never have the potential for further development.

Cognitive Dissonance and the Argument of Potentiality

In Section 1 we considered three main approaches to the question "What is the nature of a human conceptus?" One was that the conceptus is a human person. From the discussion in the previous section and some additional points made in Section 5, below, it is clear that by any definition the conceptus is not a human person. We may argue the point of its *potential* to become a human person, but at a given moment in time the *actual conceptus* is not a human person. As with any decision-making process, we must first perceive and interpret a situation based on knowledge, understanding and truth; only then can philosophical translation of events into an ethical understanding and moral teaching be possible. I submit that on the basis of what we perceive and understand by a human person—physical structure, known genetic complement, independent existence, viability, a highly coordinated network of tissues and organs, environmental and social interaction and moral status—the enigmatic conceptus, fertilized or unfertilized, is not a human person.

To be cognitive we need to be knowledgeable, to be logical rather than illogical. The so-called gut response to uncharted

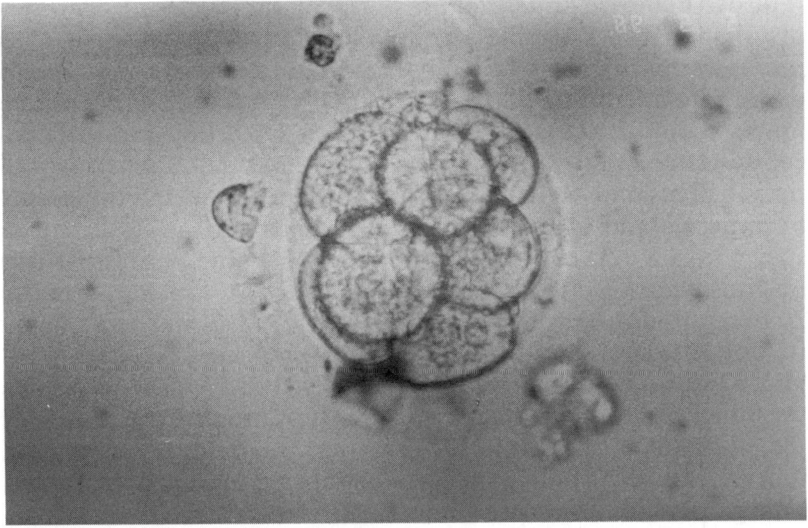

Figure 1.5

territory is understandable within limitations, but that it alone should suffice is illogical, without reason. If we were to agree that the conceptus is not actually human, then we must consider whether it is potentially human and what characteristics express this.

In the Foreword to the *Report of the Working Party Council for Science and Society*[11] Professor John Ziman stated that "society holds together by the rules that people are bound to obey. Human behavior...must always follow the constraints of biological reality. The trouble with science is that it changes biological reality. The boundary conditions on the rules of social behavior are suddenly altered, and many people become frightened." The widely applied psychological theory of cognitive dissonance demonstrates that new facts and situations must be consistent with our personal situation. If novel situations arise that are inconsistent with what we believe, dissonance results and we feel uncomfortable. Two main responses to dissonance arise: (a) an open mind is maintained, and new information is absorbed and psychological adjustment made; (b) some individuals avoid the issue entirely, refuse to believe it and develop excuses or alternatives. "Cognitive dissonance can override the human desire for truth."[12] It is precisely this response which has affected rational approaches to the nature of a human conceptus, and to preserve an inordinate moral claim on the conceptus. Those who accept that the conceptus is not a person *per se* use the argument that it is a potential person. This may be true for those conceptuses which eventually become people—but this argument may also apply to those spermatozoa and eggs which eventually become people. This is obviously not true for billions of spermatozoa, the eggs and the 70 percent of the conceptuses conceived in vivo that don't make it! The extrapolation argument, although acceptable from an end reality, is not applicable in reverse (that is, from a chance, unstable, preliminary stage) to the assumption or guarantee of the ultimate formation of human person. A fertilized egg or, indeed, the six-day-old conceptus cannot be predicted to form a human person, as nature shows us for the vast majority of conceptuses formed in vivo.[13]

It is not possible in this article to explore these arguments in depth, but from the standpoint of a scientist, I wish to look at the unusual situations arising during fertilization and cleavage and try to understand the true nature of the human conceptus.

If we consider the fertilized egg, it is a single cell with a human genetic constitution. If one is asked to list the characteristics of a person, most would think of a fully formed baby, child or adult and its responses to stimuli, apart from its obvious appearance. The conceptus would not fall into the latter category. At term we can distinguish the identity of the human person from that of any other species by simply looking at it. But the conceptuses of most mammalian species—from the mouse to the marsupials on through to man—will be indistinguishable, at least for the first week, by even the most experienced embryologist.

Observation alone is thus not a guide. What of response, or reaction to stimuli? Let us consider another single cell, the amoeba. This is an organism that exists in its fully formed state as a single cell; but this primitive creature is still more responsive to its environment than is the fertilized egg or early developing human conceptus. It moves its own mass with energy created by its own metabolism and respiration. If it approaches an undesirable area in its fluid droplet, for example, one containing an uncomfortably higher acidic content, it will hastily retreat in the opposite direction; compared to a human conceptus in such a situation, the amoeba is a highly advanced organism. But the amoeba has no potential to develop beyond its primitive state. Thus, at this early stage it is not appearance nor responsiveness to external stimuli that give us a clue to the nature of the human conceptus.

What of its genetic content? Clearly, all people have a genetic constitution that is distinctly human, and from their conception and early development, in general, they possess an identical or similar genetic constitution to that which they have as adults. So perhaps it is the genetic constitution of the conceptus that makes it a potential human person. But what of the anomalies described in Section 3? Let us look at some of those in detail.

In some nonmammalian species the embryo resulting from parthenogenetic activation, that is, the parthenogenome (or, as it is referred to in America, parthenote) can develop to a full-term individual.[14] Parthenogenesis was first referred to by Richard Owen in 1849 as "procreating without the immediate influence of a male"[15] and in 1950 by Soumalainen as "the development of the egg cell into a new individual without fertilization."[16] In mammals, types of parthenogenesis can arise, experimentally induced as well as spontaneously. Sometimes eggs can undergo parthenogenetic development into conceptuses within the ovary, as the origin of certain human and murine ovarian tumors confirms.[17] The human conceptus shown in Figure 1-6 arose without any signs of fertilization, and although appearing to be a normal, healthy, two-cell human conceptus, it is probably parthenogenetic. In some mammalian species, particularly mice, parthenogenetic development has continued to quite advanced stages after implantation, although there appears to be no potential for development to term. Clearly, this conceptus, particularly if it is diploid (having a full complement of 46 chromosomes), is not, and has no potential to be, a human person.

If two sperm enter the egg, as mentioned earlier, the resulting conceptus may be triploid. One scenario of the triploid conceptus involves its development into a conceptus that appears normal and healthy (see Figure 1.7) but may result in a partial or incomplete hydatidiform mole. If only male chromosomes remain

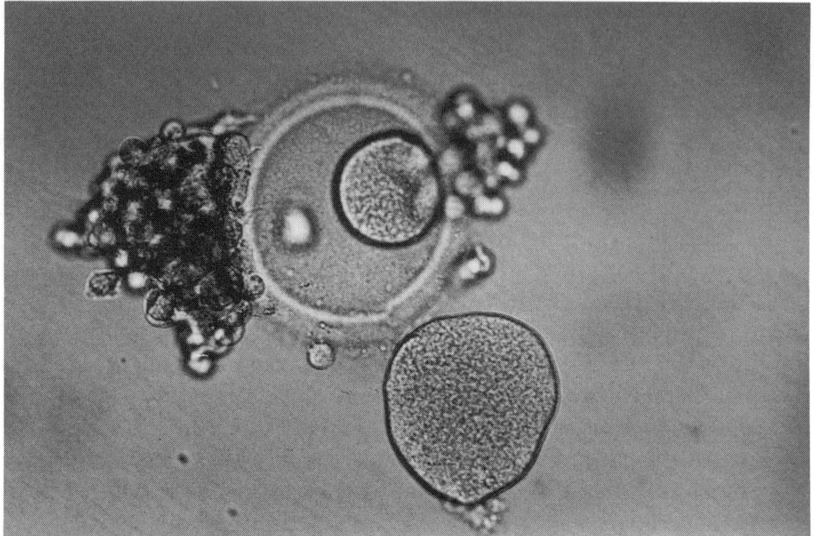

Figure 1.6

present in the conceptus—if two sperm are present and their chromosomes fuse without the female chromosomes' taking part—the conceptus will still have the normal genetic makeup of 46 chromosomes, either XX or XY, but development of this is likely to become a complete or classical hydatidiform mole. These conceptuses, therefore, develop into blastocysts that implant in the womb, but the result is haphazard placental growth and (in the case of the complete hydatidiform mole) growth with no evidence of fetal tissue and often giving rise to malignant neoplasia. From personal communication, I know of two groups practicing in-vitro fertilization that did not adequately assess the occurrence of fertilization, and their apparently normal human conceptus, after replacement into the womb, resulted in hydatidiform moles. Hence, such conceptuses are clearly not, nor do they have the potential to become, human persons.

For observation of normal fertilization of the human egg, the closely adherent follicle cells surrounding the egg must be carefully removed. This is done with fine needles, to dissect the cells away, or with very finely pulled glass pipettes so that the egg is

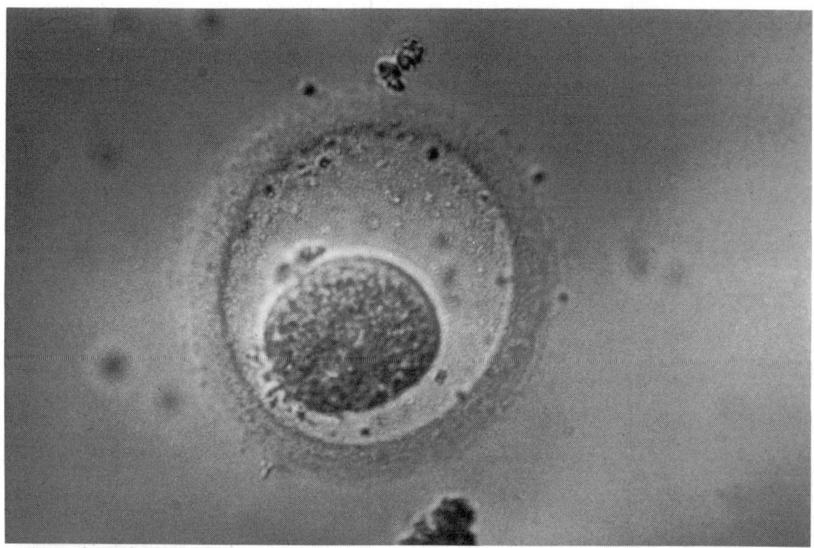

Figure 1.7

gently sucked up and down the pipette and the follicular cells eventually fall off. The technique is not without its problems. As shown in Figure 1-8, during this procedure half the cytoplasm of a fertilized egg was teased out of the zona pellucida; the result could only be a prognosis of degeneration in a short space of time (see Figure 1-9). In this situation and in any manipulation of the conceptus during the first days, if survival is impaired, what is to be the outcome if these conceptuses are considered to be people? Is the conceptus to be given a name, a death certificate and perhaps a funeral? Is it considered homicide, a crime against mankind? Surely not if it is a regular and natural occurrence for the majority of conceptuses in vivo. In Figure 1-10, the complete conceptus (with two pronuclei) burst from its zona pellucida; it developed over the next 48 hours into four separate cells (Figure 1-11). As described below, each cell is transferred to separate zonae pellucidae that could potentially develop into a set of four identical fetuses, but otherwise these have no potential for further growth. Is this homicide of one or perhaps four? Most of us who do not grant the same rights to the conceptus as a person

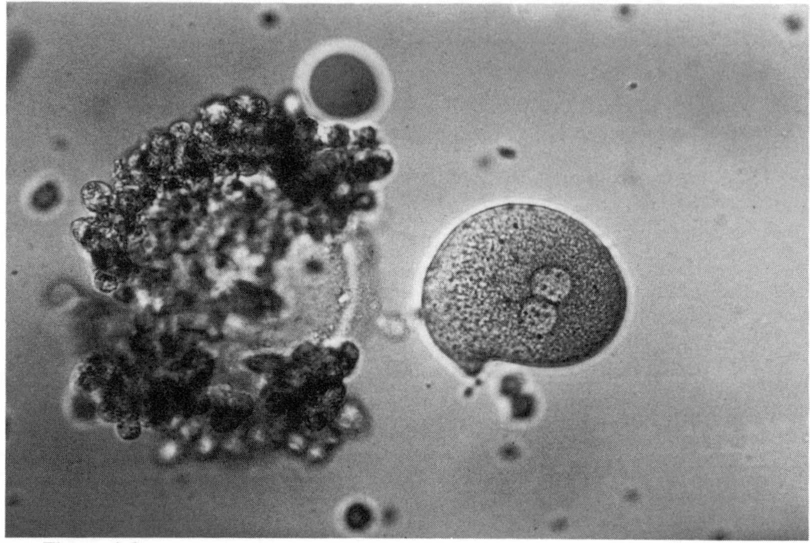

Figure 1.8

see it as an entity different from a person, a stillborn child, or even a fetus; nevertheless the conceptus may not be without a certain degree of respect and moral claim.[18]

One further consideration is related to a paper that I, with my colleagues, published in *Science* in 1983.[19] In this article we described, for the first time, the secretion of a hormone by the human conceptus. The conceptus, supernumerary to the requirements for that fertility treatment cycle, was maintained in a culture droplet for approximately 12 days after fertilization. During this time the conceptus was not interfered with except for the extraction of a small portion of the surrounding culture fluid, from which the levels of the secreted hormone were assessed; the conceptus degenerated on approximately the 12th day. After publication there followed an outcry by a certain organization, which identified this observation with murder. The important scientific message stated in the publication was that the inner ball of cells from the blastocyst, which, as stated above, would eventually become the embryo proper, actually had degenerated much earlier on, probably around the eighth day. It was the outer layer

24

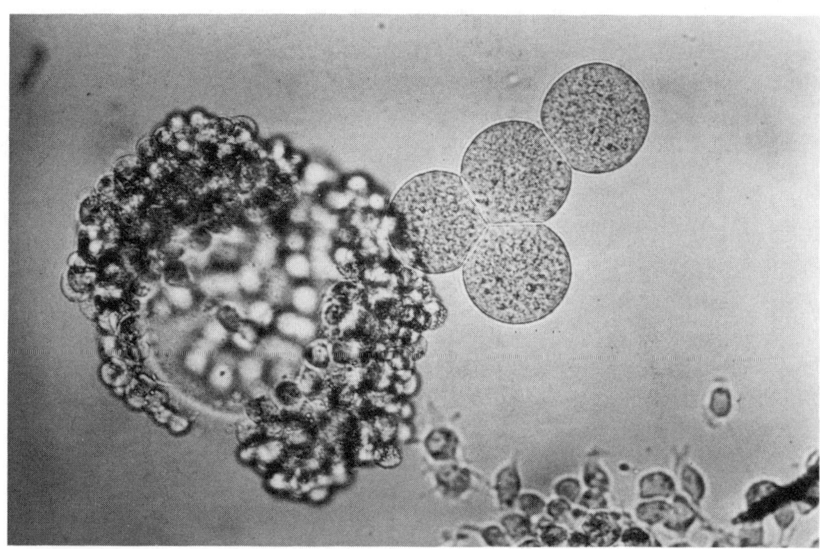

Figure 1.9

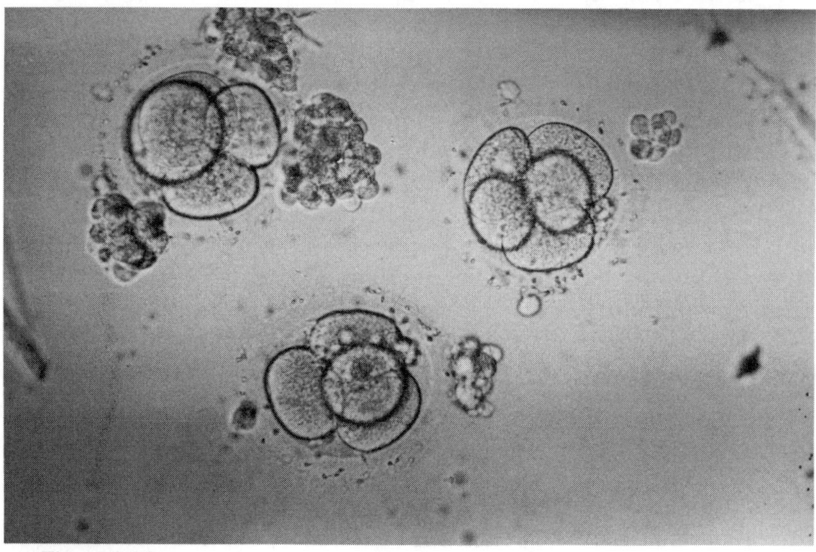

Figure 1.10

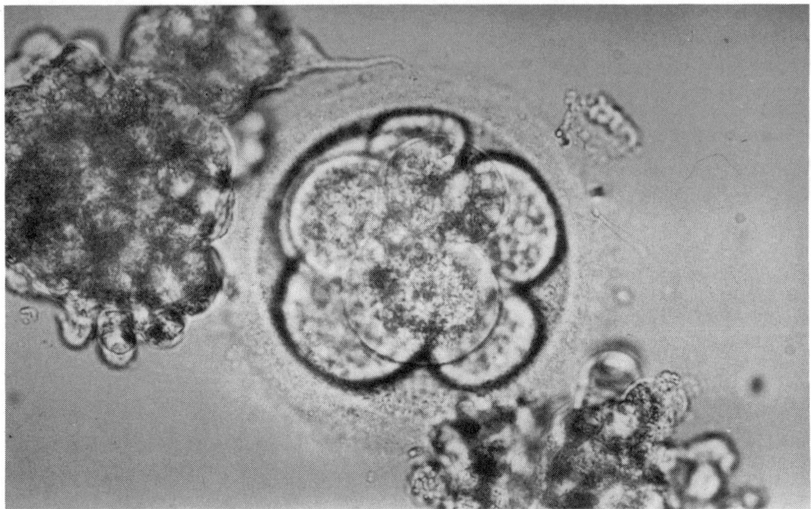

Figure 1.11

of cells that continued to grow and secrete the hormone. The outer layer of cells were destined to become only placental tissue—nothing more and with no potential of becoming a fetus. It is, in fact, the placental tissue that secretes these hormones in vivo. There is no concept of wrongdoing and no law against the study of placental cells in the amniotic fluid. Yet, because these cells were the subsequent product of an egg fertilized in vitro, cognitive dissonance resulted in an irrational, emotional reaction. Less noise is made when experimental drugs or experimental operative procedures are performed on actual adults and children—human persons as we understand them!

Birth for the Future

The birth in 1978 of the first human being conceived outside the body was a significant event, but in the professional and especially the lay community skepticism still existed. Fortunately, it was not long before this success was followed by that of the Australians. The birth, just eight years later, of more than 1,500 in-vitro fertilized children worldwide has inaugurated a new era in the treatment of infertility.

In-vitro fertilization offers a realistic opportunity for children to many couples who are sterile and to the great many who are substerile. There are few who now decry the procedure, and the majority of specialists accept in-vitro fertilization as a worthwhile procedure in the treatment of infertility.

Infertility *per se* is no longer the only domain of in-vitro fertilization. There are numerous possibilities for positive eugenics but these entail the use of gametes and pre-embryonic material. Many of the possibilities obviously require careful consideration, particularly by societies in which these techniques are perfected on animal conceptuses and where it would be a short jump to the human. In this section, we shall consider such areas as the use of freezing techniques, splitting conceptuses, chromosomal analysis in biopsied material from the conceptus, cloning, providing a donor placenta, genetic engineering and ectogenesis. Some of these are practical and "just around the corner," while others are possible but as yet not feasible.

Microinjection of sperm

Let us first consider a novel approach to a particular problem in infertility. In a significant number of couples utilizing in-vitro fertilization, penetration of the zona pellucida by a spermatozoon fails to occur. We do not yet understand the reason for the failure—whether it is a problem with the egg or the sperm. In some situations it is simply a difficulty in the binding of sperm to the egg investment and not an inherent dysfunction in either gamete. Thus, if sperm can be placed across the zona pellucida, fertilization can then occur. The technique involves micromanipulation, which has been developed for animal gametes and is being researched for human use. In the micromanipulation technique a single sperm is aspirated into a finely drawn glass pipette, which is carefully introduced through the zona pellucida, and the sperm is deposited next to the plasma membrane of the egg. The pipette is removed, and some time later the sperm fuses with the egg membrane and fertilization takes place. (See Figure 1.12)

This technique also may be used in those cases of male infertility where most sperm produced are immotile. The head of the sperm, which carries the genetic complement and the substances necessary for fertilization may still be viable although the tail is nonfunctional. In such cases, by physical transport of the sperm through the outer membrane and into the egg, fertilization is possible. Other causes of infertility that may benefit from this technique include blockage in the male reproductive tract or even an absence of the vas deferens. Spermatozoa may be aspirated from the epididymis, and although very few in number and of poor motility, these may be used to fertilize an egg by micromanipulation.

Other techniques that require micromanipulation procedures are twinning, embryonic biopsy, transfer of the inner cell mass (the embryo *per se*) to a donor trophoblastic vesicle, removal of extranumerary pronuclei, and cloning.

Twinning

As described earlier, each blastomere of the 2- or 4-cell conceptus has equal potential to undergo embryonic development to term. In animals, experiments have been done in which each blastomere of a 4-cell conceptus has been removed and placed individually in an empty zona pellucida. Various permutations have been done up to the 4-cell stage. For example, the two blastomeres of the 2-cell conceptus could be separated, or a 4-cell conceptus could be separated into two conceptuses, each having two blastomeres. In these two techniques the conceptuses, which go to cleave, would be identical twins (Figure 1-13). In the situation where a 4-cell conceptus is divided into four individual blastomeres, it is theoretically possible to achieve identical quads.

This process cannot continue indefinitely because, as mentioned previously, once the 4-cell stage has been passed, the potential for each individual blastomere to become an individual fetus is lost. The loss of this potential is, to a large extent, due to the number of cell divisions. If two blastomeres are removed from a 4-cell conceptus and allowed to divide further, the resulting conceptus will be a 4-cell. However, in terms of the number of cell divisions, because the 4-cell that it has cleaved to is by biological definition the 4-cell of an original 8-cell conceptus (that is, it has the biochemical "instincts" of an 8-cell not a 4-cell stage), it is possible to generate only identical twins or even identical quads (twinning or quadrupling!).

SPERM MICROINJECTION

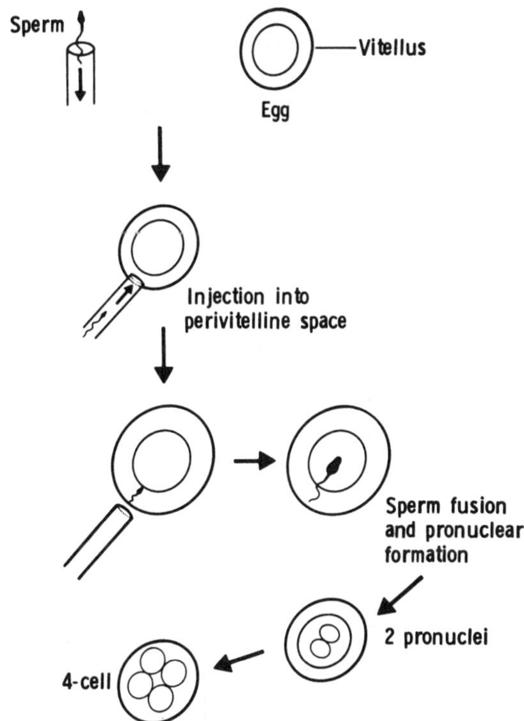

Figure 1.12

Another method of twinning has been successfully achieved in a few mammalian species, most notably farm animals. This process uses the five- or six-day conceptus, the blastocyst, or the slightly earlier stage, the morula. It is feasible to cut the blastocyst or morula literally in half, with the resultant production of two half blastocysts, each containing half an inner cell mass and trophoblast. These half blastocysts reconstitute, and although the cell number is reduced (as in the method of twinning), the potential for further development still exists (Figure 1-14).

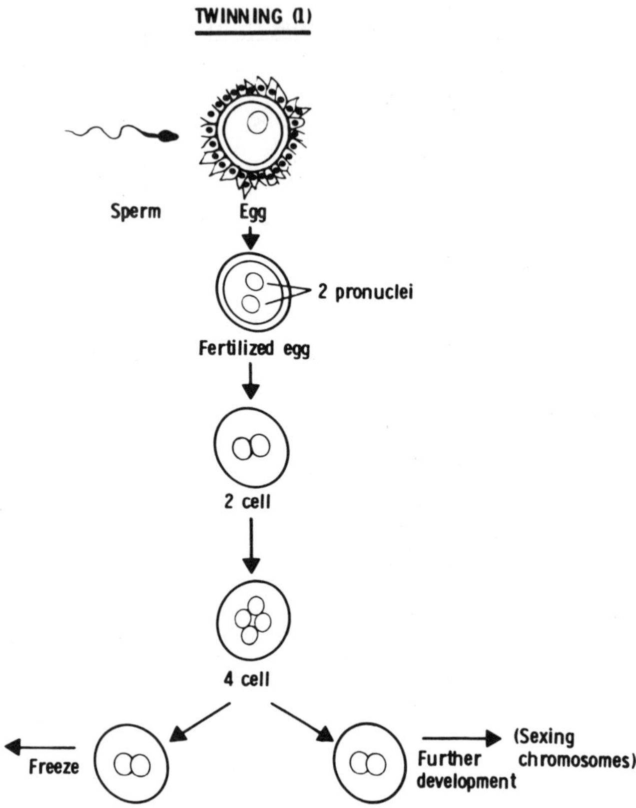

Figure 1.13

The two procedures described above are often called "cloning" because of the production of identical live young, a clone of each other. However, because of the general perceptions, the notion of cloning should be strictly reserved for the more bizarre and undesirable procedures involving the copying of an individual, that is, the cloning of a human person.

What are the advantages of twinning? As with any manipulative procedure, be it on adults or conceptuses, there should be a good clinical rationale for developing the techniques. In this instance it would be possible to examine the conceptus at these early stages for any suspected defects that may have been inherited from either or both parents. For example, if there exists a sex-linked disorder, such as hemophilia, the chromosomes of the twinned conceptus could be examined to identify its sex, and if the conceptus is male, then a decision could be made on whether or not to replace the remaining conceptus. The chromosomes could further be examined for any genetic abnormality, and with new improvements in gene probing it would be feasible to screen for genetic defects such as cystic fibrosis, Duchenne muscular dystrophy, and others. However, in all these tests, it is necessary that the conceptus be killed for the chromosomes and genes to be examined; but what is found in the twin conceptus will be an identical copy of that present in the remaining conceptus.

It is here that we see the need for clear thinking. I offer an example to highlight this point: While the Warnock Committee was gathering evidence from many representative bodies in the United Kingdom, I was fortunate to have discussions with an authority of a religious organization who, along with his religious experts, had prepared a submission to the committee. At one point the report stated categorically that "the cloning of embryonic organs for transplantation purposes is morally indefensible." The discussion on this point stipulated that cloning had to be clearly defined and that, if it were merely the removal of one or two blastomeres from a conceptus to be used for clinical investigation while the remaining conceptus still had the potential to develop to term, this should not be considered cloning in the more bizarre sense; indeed more a biopsy. Debate ensued, and in the final report submitted to Warnock, the sentence was rewritten: "The cloning of embryonic organs for transplantation purposes is morally admissible so long as this does not involve generating or cloning complete embryos for the sake of required organs." The change was made because of information gained from the nature of the conceptus and the manipulative techniques employed. An important fact in this case was that the original conceptus still had the potential to develop to term and that the manipulation was for positive eugenics, as is amniocentesis, a procedure occasionally resulting in the abortion and death of the fetus.

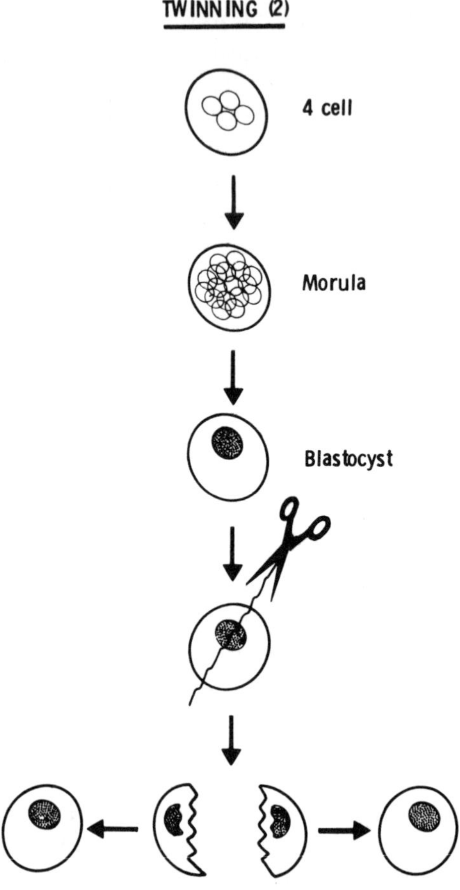

Figure 1.14

Embryonic biopsy

Somewhat different from the method of biopsy described above is a microsurgical technique more akin to biopsy as we know it. The process utilizes the blastocyst; with a very finely drawn pipette, it is possible to aspirate a few of the surrounding trophoblast cells (the precursors of the placental cells) from the blastocyst. The blastocyst *per se* can be cryopreserved, while the aspirated trophoblast cells are assessed for chromosomal or genetic defect.

Donor placenta

There is some evidence to suggest that some women who fail to have a conceptus implant or those who habitually abort have a defective placenta, caused by an incompatible trophoblast. In such circumstances it would be possible by micromanipulation to provide a donor trophoblast, that is, a donor placenta. This technique has been used successfully in animals and is similar to the twinning described above, where a donor zona pellucida is required. The technique would require the removal of the inner cell mass from one conceptus, resulting in a trophoblast vesicle (the donor trophoblast), while the inner cell mass from the union of the "parents" would be transferred to the donor trophoblast. At this stage no immunological barrier exists, and if implantation were to occur, normal development would result and the fetus would be that of the inner cell mass (Figure 1-15) of the mother carrying the child who, with her partner, are also the genetic parents.

Cryopreservation

The above-mentioned techniques would require a successful method for cryopreservation. For routine in-vitro fertilization techniques, cryopreservation offers the opportunity of storing supernumerary conceptuses (those which exceed a clinic's standard number for replacement, which varies from clinic to clinic; it is three in my clinic). These cryopreserved conceptuses may be thawed at a later date in order to achieve a pregnancy.

Cryopreservation is not yet an efficient procedure and currently may improve the incidence of success for in-vitro fertilization by only a maximum of five percent. For the microsurgical techniques mentioned above, it is imperative that efficient cryopreservation techniques be available. The twin conceptus, for example, which may eventually be replaced, will be cryopreserved in order to "mark time" while the "biopsied" cells are analyzed.

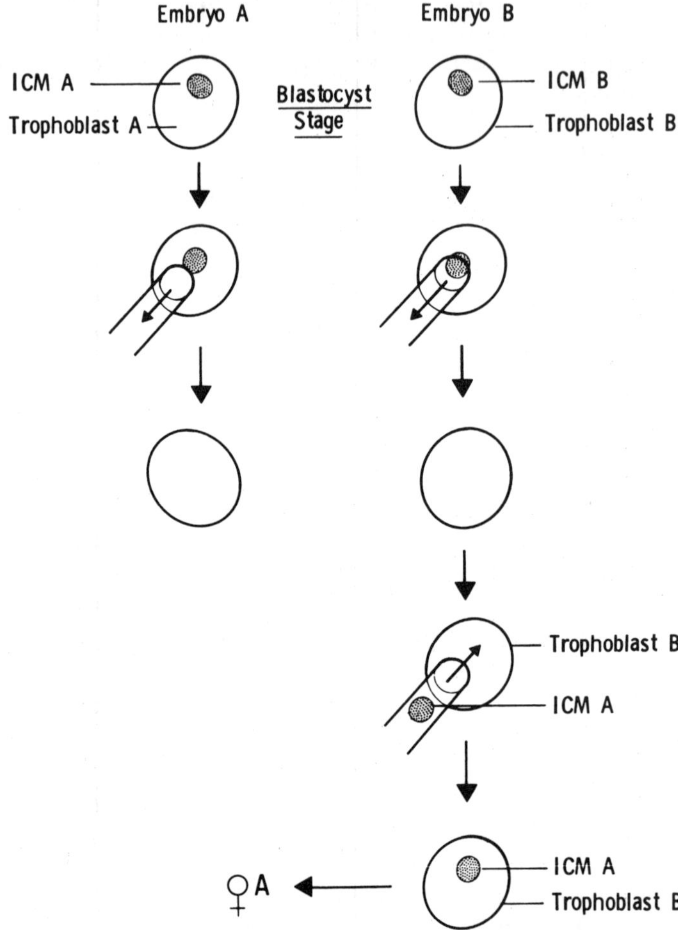

Figure 1.15

Currently, there is no human evidence to suggest that by cryopreservation of all the conceptuses obtained from a single in-vitro fertilization treatment cycle and replacement of them one or more at a time after thawing, the overall incidence of pregnancy is prejudiced. We are, therefore, rapidly approaching the situation where microsurgical biopsy and cryopreservation could be used to assess the products of conception in high risk situations.

There is a large body of literature supporting the lack of adverse effects of cryopreservation on animal conceptuses and future offspring. It also appears that this conclusion is applicable to human beings although fewer than 100 children have been born by this method so far. This may not be the situation for the cryopreservation of eggs, where the chromosomes are at a more "delicate" stage of cell division, compared to the conceptus. So far it has proved more difficult to cryopreserve the egg, and for the reasons stated much work needs to be done to assess the safety of this technique. However, many would find it ethically more acceptable to store the unfertilized egg than the conceptus, but currently it is biologically more difficult to justify.

Removal of extranumerary pronuclei

It was mentioned earlier that for various reasons—more than one sperm's entering the egg or failure of extrusion of the second polar body after fertilization—the fertilized egg may have more than two pronuclei. With microsurgical techniques it is possible, at least in some conceptuses, to distinguish the male from the female pronucleus. It may be feasible to remove one of the extra pronuclei in the three-pronucleate egg, which will permit the conceptus to resume a normal diploid state and thereby develop normally. This would be a very useful procedure if, for example, after in-vitro fertilization the patient had only three eggs and two or three contained more than two pronuclei. If more than one conceptus is replaced after in-vitro fertilization, the incidence of pregnancy is significantly increased (from 10 to 45 percent for one to three conceptuses in my clinic). Hence, the ability to remove extranumerary pronuclei and permit the patient to receive three apparently normal conceptuses would be of great benefit in establishing a pregnancy. It also would permit the correction of a defective fertilization.

Nuclear substitution of cloning

Cloning is a technique often associated with the bizarre and horrendous ideas of "*The Boys from Brazil.*"[20] It is interesting that few would object on ethical grounds to the formation of identical twins, as they are a natural phenomenon. Yet, these are a clone of each other. But the abhorrence at the cloning of an infant, adolescent, or adult would be universal. Perhaps it is because the latter are recognized as members of the community, human persons, as opposed to the conceptus, whose developmental scenario is incomplete. This is not to say that a child's developmental scenario is complete, but society already has recognized its existence with a birth certificate.

To achieve this form of cloning (to make an identical copy of a person), it would be necessary to transplant that person's complete genetic constitution into a fertilized egg. A theoretical approach to this would be to take a nucleus from a person's somatic cell and remove the pronuclei from a fertilized human egg and replace these with the somatic nucleus. This would have the effect of introducing that person's genetic constitution into the fertilized (activated) egg, which may then cleave and develop according to the introduced genetic makeup (Figure 1-16). If this egg developed to term, it would be an identical copy (a clone) of that person. However, evidence from experiments on some mammalian conceptuses suggests that, in the foreseeable future at least, the success of this technique is inconceivable. The biological circumstances are so unlikely that it would be unreasonable to be seriously concerned about such a fanciful speculation.

Ectogenesis

It is also fanciful speculation to consider the prolonged development, especially to term, of a conceptus outside the womb. By a conservative estimate, fewer than 20 percent and probably fewer than 10 percent of human conceptuses fertilized in vitro will develop to the six- or seven-day blastocyst and "hatch" from the zona pellucida. Optimal culture conditions, that is, milieu analogous to the conditions in the Fallopian tube and uterus, are unknown. The period of implantation is a particularly difficult biological constraint. Under current knowledge, it is difficult to imagine successful development in vitro through 14 days of post-fertilization, let alone further development. However, more conceptuses reaching the blastocyst stage could be obtained if the conceptuses were first fertilized in vivo and, by uterine lavage, collected and further cultured in vitro.

NUCLEAR TRANSFERS
Sperm
Egg A
Egg B
Somatic cell
Nucleus
2 pronuclei
Egg A
fertilized
Egg B
fertilized
Removal of
somatic
nucleus
Removal of
♀ pronuclei
Removal of
♂ and ♀
pronuclei
Enucleated
fertilized
egg
Transfer of
somatic nucleus
to fertilized
enucleated egg
?
4 cell
Fusion of ♂ (A)
and ♀ (B) pronuclei
CLONE

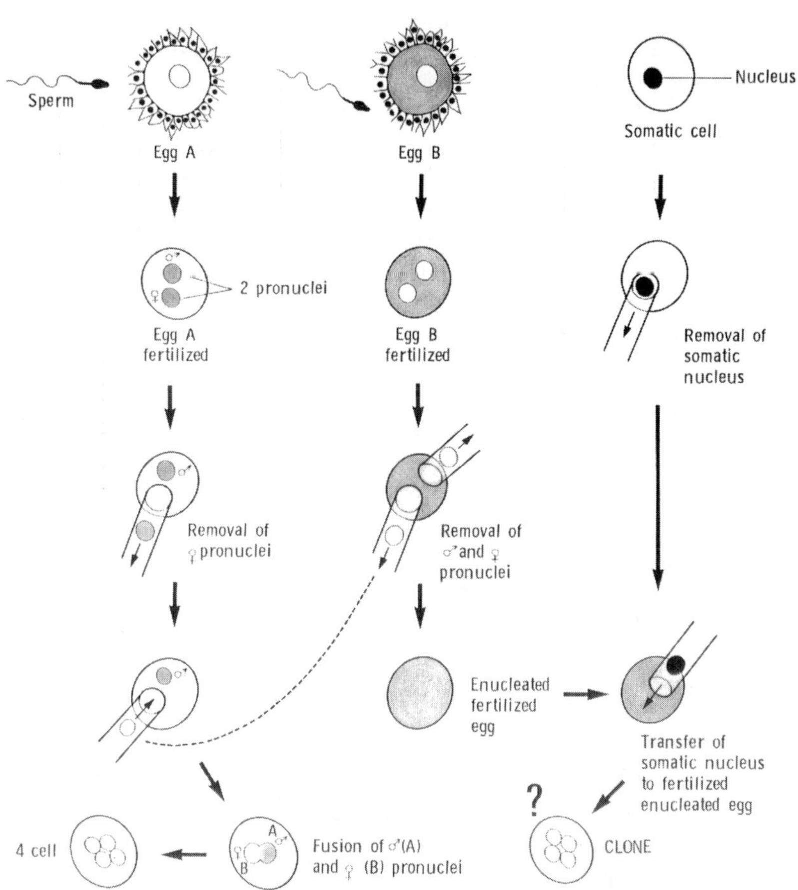

Figure 1.16

Even mice conceptuses, of which 95 percent may reach the blastocyst stage in vitro, have proved extremely difficult to grow beyond the early implantation stage. The process of implantation *per se* presents enormous biological barriers, although later stages removed from the womb have developed for a few days. However, to consider ectogenesis from the conceptus to term would seem highly unlikely with current knowledge.

Nevertheless, some development of the human conceptus in vitro, if ever achieved, could be used to study the abnormal as well as the normal stages of early human development. It also would permit the opportunity to investigate the effect of drugs that, as thalidomide, have specific effects on the human fetus. Most professional bodies wish to see guidelines on the maximum period of growth outside the body ranging from 14 to 30 days. By days 22 and 23 after fertilization the neural folds, which eventually fuse, appear in the embryo, and by day 30 the recognizable antecedent of the spinal cord is present.

At this point, it is interesting to note that a spontaneously aborted surviving fetus is given every advanced medical aid to keep it alive; many at 28 weeks now survive. The conceptus, however, clearly perceived differently, is not permitted this attention: the provision of an artificial environment to promote further development if no womb is available. Indeed, the Warnock Report wishes it to be deemed a criminal offense to prolong the existence of the in-vitro conceptus beyond 14 days—it must be killed!

Gene therapy

Correcting a disorder by the direct injection into the nuclear material of the actual gene that codes for the correct version of an anomalous protein is an idea that has been around for some time. The gene for growth hormones has been injected into mice conceptuses and this has been incorporated into the embryonic DNA, resulting in extra production of growth hormone; after such conceptuses had been implanted into recipient females, some developed to term and resulted in giant-sized mice.

The possibility of correcting certain genetic disorders—for example, injecting the normal insulin allele if the natural one is defective—at the embryonic stage must be considered realistic. Although such therapy would, in theory, be a great step toward positive eugenics, many technical difficulties exist: The defective or absent gene first must be detected; a healthy gene for injection also must be available; the technique must cause minimal damage to each cell. But even if each of these conditions were met, it is not yet possible to ensure that the gene will be successfully incorporated into the host genome, will be transcribed correctly, and will ultimately produce a normal protein. There are many risks with such a procedure, and an enormous amount of work on animal cells and/or conceptuses first must be done to ensure safety and efficacy. It will be many years before a number of human genes are available for such use.

A more realistic approach for the future would be to attempt to obtain a healthy colony of cells in vitro (perhaps with embryonic cells for transplantation—see below) and use these to colonize an adult suffering from a particular disorder. Perhaps defective cells from the adult could be recovered, corrected by gene therapy, tested, and allowed to proliferate further in vitro before being returned to the host. For embryonic material, in the near future it would be more realistic and safer to concentrate on techniques for the detection of defects and subsequent abortion in vitro, as described above.

Embryonic cells for transplantation

Embryonic and early stage fetal cells do not possess a trait characteristic of later fetal and adult cells. The latter have the ability to induce an immune reaction when transplanted into an adult host; the former do not. Experiments with animals demonstrate the advantage early fetal cells have in colonizing the host. Cultured fetal mouse pancreatic cells, when transplanted, can successfully colonize a diabetic splenectomized, adult host mouse and reverse the diseased state of the adult. It may be possible, for example, that the hemopoietic cells (precursors of the blood cells) of the postimplantation human embryo could be injected into children or adults with lethal blood diseases. Early embryonic cells (up to 20 days after fertilization) should be considered usable for such prospects within the next decade.

Concluding Remarks

I have attempted to highlight some of the main areas of current research on the human conceptus and some research that may be developed in the near future. I have also mentioned some of the more fanciful and impractical ideas about which many people are concerned. All such research, however, cannot be considered as isolated scientific studies by a few rather "odd, irresponsible scientists." The research achieved yesterday, today, and tomorrow is along the path that has been and will be laid down by the inquiring mind of the human species. All research associated with human conceptuses or pre-embryonic material must be considered with a clear perception of the nature of the human conceptus and the nature of the research. Consequently, I have tried to place the research in this context.

Centuries of knowledge have changed our views and the world in which we live. Mankind cannot avoid change, and society cannot afford to ignore knowledge, the pursuit of which is the nature of *Homo sapiens*. The accumulation of knowledge in the key areas of science and medicine that led to the birth of the first human conceived extracorporeally is an example of mankind's progressive collaborative skills. The need for the knowledge of human reproduction to be put into a realistic context, to permit moral and ethical judgments, has been discussed. Once we *understand* what is being done, what it is possible to do, and for what purpose we should do research, then we can judge what should be done.

NOTES

This chapter was originally written for the ICUS Conference in Washington in November 1986 and represents the state of In-vitro research up to that date.

1. *Report of the Committee of Enquiry into Human Fertility and Embryology*, cmnd. 9314. (London: HMSO, 1984).
2. W.T. Smith, "On a New Method of Treating Sterility by the Removal of Obstructions of the Fallopian Tubes," *Lancet* 1 (1849), 603.
3. W. L. Estes, Jr., and P. L. Heitmeyer, "Pregnancy Following Ovarian Implantation," *Amer. J. Surg.* 24 (1934), 563.

4. S. L. Schnek, "Das Sagethieri kunstlich befruchtet ausserhalb des Mutterthieres," *Mitt. Embryolog,* Inst. Univ. Wien 2 (1878), 107.

5. G. Pincus, and E. B. Enzman, "Can Mammalian Eggs Undergo Normal Development In-vitro?" *Proc. Nat. Acad. Sci.* 20 (1934), 121.

6. N. F. Menkin, and J. Rock, "In-vitro Fertilization and Cleavage of Human Ovarian Eggs," *Amer. J. of Obstet. Gyn.* 55 (1948), 440.

7. L. B. Shettles, "The Living Human Ovum," *Amer. J. Obstet. Gyn.* 76 (1958), 398.

8. F. Bacon. *Novum organum* (London: 1620).

9. K. Edmonds, K. Lindsay, J. Miller, E. Williamson and P. Wood, "Early Embryonic Mortality in Women," *Fertil. Steril.* 38 (1983), 447.

10. T. J. Hassold, and A. Matsuyama, "Origin of Trisomes in Human Spontaneous Abortions," *Human Genet.* 46 (1978), 285.

11. John Ziman, "Human Procreation: Ethical Aspects of the New Techniques," in *Report of the Working Party Council for Science and Society* (Oxford: Oxford, 1984).

12. M. Ben Yosef, and G. Robinson, *The 2001 Principle* (Jerusalem: Hed, 1983).

13. See reference 9.

14. U. Mittwoch, "Panthenogenesis," *J. Med. Genet.* 15 (1978), 165.

15. R. Owen, *On Parthenogenesis, or the Successive Production of Procreating Individuals from a Single Ovum* (London: Little, van Voorst, 1849).

16. E. Suomalinen, "Parthenogenesis in Animals." *Advan. Genet.* 3 (1950), 193.

17. D. Lynder, B. K. McCaw, and F. Hecht, "Parthenogenetic Origin of Benign Ovarian Teratomas." *New Eng. J. Med.* 292 (1975), 63.

18. G. Dunstan, "Human In-vitro Fertilization: The Ethical Debate," in S. Fishel and E. M. Symonds, (eds.), *Human In-vitro Fertilization: Past, Present, Future* (Oxford: IRL, 1986).

19. S. B. Fishel, R. G. Edwards and C. J. Evans, "Human Chorionic Gonatropin Secreted by Pre-implantation Embryos Cultured In-vitro," *Science* 223 (1984), 816.

20. I. Levin, *The Boys From Brazil* (London: Pan, 1977).

GLOSSARY

Amniocentesis. The insertion of a needle into the amniotic cavity (the fluid-filled sac surrounding the fetus) to remove some of the fluid and the exfoliated cells. These cells can be assessed for the sex of the fetus or any genetic abnormality. The fluid also may be assessed for any abnormality.

Androgenome. A conceptus or fetus developing solely with male (paternal) genes. There are no heritable characteristics passed on from the female.

Asthenospermia. The production of normal numbers of spermatozoa in the ejaculate but with a high percentage immotile.

Blastocyst. The stage of the conceptus in which it becomes a large spherical structure with a centralized fluid-filled cavity. It is at this stage that two cell types first form in the conceptus: the trophoblasts, which are the precursor cells to the placenta and surround the edge of the blastocyst, and the inner cell mass which is a ball of cells at one pole of the blastocyst and will eventually differentiate into the embryo proper. This stage arises approximately five days after fertilization.

Endometriosis. Isolated pockets of tissue from the lining of the womb occurring at other sites, for example, the ovary, the Fallopian tubes and the cervix. The specific connection of this condition with fertility is unknown, but its association with infertility is established.

Epigenesis. The development of an organism from an undifferentiated cell; or developmental direction's being organized by external causal factors rather than intrinsic preformation.

Female antisperm antibodies. Produced by the female antibodies against spermatozoa: These antibodies will attack and immobilize spermatozoa from any male and are not specific to an individual.

Gynogenome. The result of the development of a conceptus or fetus without the occurrence of fertilization.

Hydatidiform mole. A fleshy mass formed in the uterus by the degeneration or abortive development of an ovum. This development appears as an abnormal pregnancy; a mass of cysts resembling a bunch of grapes appears in the uterine cavity.

Induced male infertility. The production of antibodies by an individual male antisperm autoantibodies against his own spermatozoa.

Laparoscope. An instrument like a telescope for insertion through the navel to visualize the abdominal cavity.

Morula. The stage in the development of the conceptus in which the individual cells fuse together and form a united mass, each cell being inseparable from another. This occurs about four days after fertilization.

Oligospermia. The production of small numbers of spermatozoa in the ejaculate.

Parthenogenesis. The development of a conceptus or fetus without fertilization.

Premature menopause. A condition in which the ovaries cease to function and become depleted of their primary follide store before the age at which the menopause occurs naturally. Arbitrarily set at 35 years.

Splenectomyzed. The removal of the spleen.

Teratospermia. The production of normal numbers of spermatozoa with good motility but with a high percentage of abnormal appearance.

Vasa deferentia. The canals that carry the spermatozoa from the testicles to the penis.

TWO

THE VALUE Of IN-VITRO RESEARCH

Robert Winston

In-vitro fertilization (IVF) and embryo research has significantly improved our understanding and treatment of the infertile. Infertility is a huge human problem. One in 10 of all couples are affected by it. Because it is so common, it causes human distress more frequently than any other affliction. It has occupied man's attention since time immemorial. It is no accident that the Bible is literally packed with examples of the effects of infertility. No fewer than three out of the four matriarchs suffered the pain of childlessness. Rachel says to her husband, Jacob, (Genesis 30:1) "Havah lee vonim, ve'im ayin-mathai anouchi"—"Give me children, or if not, I am dead." One famous medieval commentator, Rabbi Solomon ben Isaac of Troyes, annotates "I am dead" as "dead of grief and shame." With great insight, Genesis tells us that Jacob turned to Rachel angrily at her statement, eloquently demonstrating the friction between man and wife that sterility provokes. Why should Rachel, the favorite wife, Jacob's first choice, the most beautiful and given all gifts, have felt so bitter that she wished to die? It is because she had lost her self-esteem, her status. Sarah, in similar distress, tells her husband, Abraham, to have a child by Hagar, her handmaiden (Genesis 16:2) "oolai ibonay mimano"—"that I may be builded up through her."

Infertility erodes the most basic of human feelings. Couples often initially experience sadness, followed by anger, shame or guilt. For many, it leads to a deep threat to their sexuality; men frequently become impotent and women anorgasmic. The marital recrimination and disharmony that follow may lead to divorce, depression and a feeling of the meaninglessness of life itself. Why should infertility, not a life-threatening condition in the accepted sense, pose such a deep threat? This distinguished audience should perhaps be reminded that, no matter how successful we are in other walks of life, we leave remarkably little behind us. Should we even gain a Nobel Prize, within a matter of 15 years or less, our achievements might justify a footnote in eight-point type at the bottom of a page of a large textbook. The most we can usually hope is that we produce children to contribute to succeeding generations.

Research on human embryos already has alleviated some of this suffering. As a result of this work, we now understand far more about the various causes of sub-fertility. It also led directly to the development of a revolutionary therapy—IVF. Without embryo research, the 2,000 healthy babies already born as a result of this treatment would not exist. One patient of mine recently confronted her Member of Parliament outside the House of Commons in Westminster. She asked him why he had consistently promoted a bill devised to ban all embryo research. He replied by saying that he was opposed to the destruction of human life. Thereupon, she lifted her IVF baby from the pram and said, "Do you call this destruction of human life?"

Although IVF has been developed, it is still largely very unsuccessful. In the U.K. so far, less than 1,000 babies have been born after this procedure—yet more than 500,000 British couples are infertile. Seen in this light, many improvements are urgently needed. IVF remains the least successful of all infertility procedures, but it has a high profile. Each day, the press still claims "New Hopes for Childless Couples." In many ways, the charisma surrounding IVF has diverted the attention of fertility specialists and their patients from more pressing needs. IVF remains the most complex, expensive and emotionally demanding of all infertility treatments. Paradoxically, it is still the least successful. Dr. Trounson is correct when he points out that the global significance of IVF is as yet minuscule in clinical terms.

Apart from the management of infertility, there are numerous other potential benefits to be derived from embryo research. Miscarriage is depressingly common. Perhaps 15 percent of human pregnancies abort spontaneously. At least 100,000 women in the U.K. and 500,00 women in the U.S.A. miscarry annually. Apart from the costs of admitting such women to hospitals, miscarriage is a severe emotional shock—an event that lives with many women years after the loss of the life within the uterus. Moreover, miscarriage can result in permanent damage to the genital tract and, for a few women, especially in countries with more primitive medical services, it is life-threatening. Although we appreciate now that many miscarriages occur because the fetus is chromosomally defective, the exact genesis of miscarriage is quite mysterious. Doctors are quite unable to explain to most patients why they have lost their early pregnancy. Because many miscarriages are likely to be due to defective embryogenesis, it follows that research on embryos could provide important insights into the precise aetiology of this important condition.

Ectopic pregnancy, when the fetus implants outside the womb, is also common. About 1 in every 150 pregnancies in Europe is ectopic. In some countries, such as Jamaica, the incidence of ectopic pregnancy is 10 times more common. Ectopic pregnancy causes massive abdominal hemorrhage and most sufferers require major emergency abdominal surgery to save their lives. In many countries, ectopic pregnancy is a significant cause of maternal death. Why the fetus should implant in this way is unknown. Research into human embryonic implantation is almost certainly the only way to provide a real insight into this disease. Animal embryo research is largely useless, as no mammal other than the human is prone to extra-uterine implantation.

Contraception is recognized as a major global problem. Perhaps, if we do not destroy ourselves with nuclear weapons during the next 20 years, overpopulation presents the greatest threat to human well-being. Without exception, existing contraceptive methods are unpopular with a substantial proportion of the world's population, either because of side-effects, or because particular methods cause religious or social difficulties. For example, sterilization is poorly accepted partly because it leaves a physical scar which is unwelcome in many societies or because it is largely irreversible. We need methods of contraception which either prevent fertilization or which stops early embryos from growing. Whatever compounds are discovered, it is essential that they are tested first with human embryonic material. Only this will ensure that, in the event of failure of the method, there is no risk of an abnormal baby developing.

The problems of genetic defect, above all, lead researchers to wish to study embryo development. Although much of this work initially has been done using animal models, the study of human material will be essential. Animal embryos develop differently and each mammalian species has unique features. Animals do not develop the same genetic defects as humans; for example, monkeys do not produce babies suffering from Down's Syndrome. About 14,000 babies each year in the United Kingdom die as a result of birth defect—the second most common cause of infant death after prematurity. Many more survive for a time, or lead hopelessly inhumane lives, until diseases such as pneumonia catch up with them and they die. The disruption and cost to the families of these children is horrendous.

One curious fact is that our own society has completed accepted methods of contraception which destroy quite advanced embryos. We also encourage termination of pregnancy when the fetus is deformed. Yet, the British Parliament recently has shown great hesitation in allowing embryo research to establish methods to detect genetic defect. If this work comes to fruition, as seems probable, then the need for some abortions (which destroy fully-formed fetuses) will become unnecessary—doctors will simply be able to take several embryos simultaneously from a couple and, after a biopsy, place only those into the uterus which can be shown to be healthy.

At least 10 percent of human diseases are genetically determined. Once molecular biological techniques are applied to embryo research, we shall develop enormous potential for dealing with many serious illnesses. Of course, our society must control this work. Genetic manipulation clearly has great potential for evil as well as good. The next stage in man's development may be the genesis of advanced, superhuman computers. An alternative, no less threatening, is the possibility that man contrives genetic techniques which hasten evolution. History shows that scientific progress is never halted. It is up to us to insure that embryo research does not destroy or damage human life, but that it continues to be used to promote and protect it.

THREE

CHRISTIAN BELIEF and The ETHICS Of IN-VITRO FERTILIZATION RESEARCH

Paul Badham

Most pressure groups campaigning for a ban on in-vitro research and for the repeal of "liberal" abortion laws are self-consciously Christian. But can they legitimately claim the support of the Christian heritage for their position? This paper details Christian criticisms of seemingly comparable medical innovations in the past and notes that few Christians today would wish to endorse such opposition. The case of in-vitro fertilization research may not exactly parallel those earlier medical advances, however, because there is an additional crucial argument. The central claim made by Christian critics is that personhood exists from the moment of conception, and hence, even at its earlier stages of development, the embryo should be seen as sacrosanct. This claim is tested against the witness of the Bible, the traditions of the Church, and the requirements of Christian reasoning. The conclusion is that no adequate foundation exists for this viewpoint to be proclaimed as "the Christian position."

In-vitro research has immense positive possibilities. One of the greatest blessings of human life is the "heritage and the gift of children,"[1] and this is something that in-vitro research already has given to many formerly childless couples. It was a joyful and natural human instinct that led the future Pope John Paul I to welcome so warmly the birth of the first test tube baby[2] before further consideration of the issues involved led his church to a more negative stance towards such research. Yet, the restoration of hope to barren couples is only the first of many good things that in-vitro research may bring. It also offers the possibility of reducing or eliminating some of the terrible handicaps that can be passed on through genetic defect, and it offers the potential of a deeper understanding of the workings of the human organism and hence the possibility of a future cure or prevention of some forms of d isease.[3] Hence, as Cardinal Basil Hume has written, if the question were considered "solely in utilitarian terms," everyone would be in favor of the continuation of such experiments. However, the Cardinal believes that, if consideration were to be given to the "absolute moral values" inherent in the "Judeo-Christian tradition," a very different conclusion would be reached.[4] And in this, Basil Hume speaks for much Christian opinion; for many of the pressure groups campaigning against the continuation of in-vitro research do so from avowedly Christian premises.[5] Thus, although working parties of moral theologians and scientists set up by the churches sometimes have been favorably disposed toward continuation of such research,[6] Christian opinion at a grass-roots level seems strongly opposed to it; and such opposition is also the present unequivocal stance of the Roman Catholic and Orthodox churches.[7]

Turning to the analogous issue of abortion, we face a comparable situation. On the one hand, many countries have adopted "liberal" abortion laws, which enjoy a fair measure of popular support. On the other hand, such reforms, though sometimes supported by liberal theologians and even by quasi-official Anglican or Protestant commissions,[8] are bitterly opposed by a groundswell of ordinary Christian opinion in all churches, as well as by the official teaching of the Roman Catholic and Orthodox churches. In Britain, for example, most women now want the present law to stay[9] while, by contrast, explicitly Christian opinion has swung dramatically against it. Thus, although the British Abortion Act of 1967 closely followed the recommendations made in 1965 by the Church of England's Board for Social Responsibility, Anglican opinion has changed so dramatically since then that the General Synod now wants the law to be radically amended, and has affirmed by a majority of 256 votes to 2 that "life developing in the womb is created by God in his own image, and is, therefore, to be nurtured, supported and protected."[10]

Hence, on both in-vitro research and abortion a clear difference of opinion appears to exist between utilitarian, or pragmatic, secular thought and the views of many contemporary Christians. This difference is important because the continuation of both in-vitro research and of liberal abortion laws are at risk at the present time. Already in-vitro research is very restricted in the United States, while in Britain two attempts to prohibit it altogether have been headed off only by Parliamentary filibustering. Liberal abortion laws still are attacked bitterly in several European countries, and in the United States, a change of personnel in the Supreme Court might well remove the constitutional defense of women's "right to choose." Already Congress has banned federal medical aid for abortions for the poor, while the Administration now denies funds to any Third World aid agency that encourages abortion, thereby reducing its availability in precisely those areas most at risk from overpopulation and famine. It is apparent that "the Catholic Church and the fundamentalist Protestant religions form the backbone of the anti-abortion movement,"[11] as well as spearheading the onslaught against in-vitro research. I want, therefore, to explore the grounds on which many Christians claim that their opposition is a necessary or inevitable part of an authentically Christian outlook.

Historical Comparisons

I am prompted to question this Christian position not the least because, as a church historian, I am very conscious of how Christians of previous ages have denounced vehemently medical practices that no Christian today would dream of rejecting. For centuries Christian opinion forbade the giving of medicine,[12] the practice of surgery, the study of anatomy, or the dissection of corpses for medical research. Later, the practices of inoculation and vaccination faced fierce theological condemnation, as did the initial use of quinine against malaria.[13] The introduction of anesthesia and, above all, the use of chloroform in childbirth were seen as directly challenging the divine edict that "in pain you shall bring forth children,"[14] and hence were violently denounced from public pulpits throughout Britain and the United States.[15] But today, there can be few Christians who would seriously question the morality of surgery, anatomical research or anesthesia. Yet, many of the arguments used against in-vitro research today are similar to those formerly employed against the medical innovations of earlier ages.[16] Accusations of "playing God," of unwillingness to accept that God knows best what is right for a particular person, of failing to appreciate the dignity of the human body made in the image of God, or of prying into the sacred mysteries were brought routinely against the first students of anatomy and against those who sought to combat the onslaught of disease or suffering by surgery, newly-discovered drugs or anesthesia.[17]

It seems that there is a strong tendency for believers in a divine providence to oppose innovations in medical practice as implying a lack of faith and trust in God's good purposes. Yet, after the medical practice in question has become common, opposition tends to fade, and the formerly criticized activity of the doctor comes to be perceived as being in itself a channel of God's sustaining love and as the vehicle of his sustaining providence. Consequently, although the practice of medicine had to fight bitter ecclesiastical opposition in early centuries, a very close relationship often now exists between doctors and clergy,[18] and medically-trained Christian missionaries have made a substantial contribution to the worldwide diffusion of Western medicine. It is therefore possible that, if in-vitro research is permitted to continue and if much observable good follows from it, the present Christian outcry against it may gradually fade, and like other medical techniques it may come to be seen as a God-given gift to the human race. Indeed, I have already heard a grateful mother, speaking on a radio program about her experience with medically-assisted fertilization, describe it as a "gift from heaven."[19]

However, a change of this kind in the prevailing Christian attitude may not necessarily happen because one key argument, used against both in-vitro fertilization and abortion, is substantially different from the arguments used against earlier medical innovations: that from the moment of conception the pre-embryo is a human being, and therefore as much entitled to protection and care as any adult person. This claim is the foundation of the "absolutist" case against both abortion and in-vitro fertilization research, on the grounds that the fetus is a person and hence that destroying it is equivalent to murder.

The dating of personhood from the moment of conception enjoys substantial support across a wide spectrum of the Christian community nowadays; indeed, many see it as axiomatic that a committed Christian will, because of this dating, wish to ban in-vitro research and repeal existing abortion legislation. What I wish to do is to question the validity of such an assumption and explore whether Christian belief necessarily entails the view that a fetus in the earliest stages of its development should be regarded as already a person.

My starting point will be the premise that a belief cannot be regarded as distinctly *Christian* unless it can be shown to be based on the teaching of the Scriptures, the tradition of the Church through the ages, and the requirements of an informed reason working today within the framework of faith. This does not imply any spirit of either biblical or ecclesiastical fundamentalism—as if Christians today were bound to share all the beliefs of their long-dead predecessors. But it *does* suggest that, if there is any sense in which Christianity can be regarded as a "revealed" religion, there must be in the sources of Christian belief some foundation for any opinion that is to be put forward as characteristic of an authentically Christian outlook. On this premise, let us therefore examine the opinion that an embryo is human, a person.

The Teaching of the Bible

The Bible certainly teaches the value of human life[20] and forbids the murder of any human being. But in biblical terms, life commences only when the breath enters the nostrils; then man or woman becomes "a living being,"[21] and this has consistently been taught in the Jewish tradition since biblical times.[22] Consequently, in biblical terms the fetus is not a person. This is brought out clearly in the laws relating to murder. For though the Ten Commandments in Exodus, Chapter 20, state clearly, "You shall not murder," in the following chapter the text goes on to differentiate between causing the death of an adult human being and causing the death of an unborn fetus. For whereas "Whoever hits a man and kills him is to be put to death,"[23] "If some men are fighting and hurt a pregnant woman so that she loses her child, but is not injured in any other way, the one who hurt her is to be fined."[24] There is no suggestion in the Old Testament law, as there is in a comparable Assyrian one, that "he who struck her shall compensate for her fetus with a life."[25] Indeed, the biblical text does not even regard the loss of her fetus as causing the woman harm; for it goes on to specify what should happen "if any harm follows."[26] At no point is any consideration given to the notion that the fetus itself might be thought to have rights. And this absence of concern for the fetus is also implied by the imposition of the death penalty on women who conceive out of wedlock, without any consideration being given to the fact that this penalty killed both the fetus and the woman.[27]

Turning to the issue of abortion as such, I am somewhat puzzled that biblical fundamentalists, who oppose abortion so strongly, should pay so little heed to the silence of the Bible. It is usually dangerous to imply that "silence gives consent"; nevertheless, the silence is surprising, given that the deliberate causing of a miscarriage seems to be referred to in ancient Sumerian, Assyrian, Babylonian, Hittite, and Persian laws,[28] and as we have already seen, the Assyrian law states quite categorically that killing a fetus is equivalent to homicide.[29] Since the Old Testament drew upon "a common background of legal jurisprudence shared throughout much of the ancient Near East,"[30] it is noteworthy that no identification of abortion with homicide is made in the

Old Testament, even though many other ancient laws were incorporated, albeit in modified form. But whether this silence is significant or not, the fact ought to be faced that, whatever views one may hold about abortion, no straightforward appeal can be made to the teaching of the Bible; for the Bible simply does not discuss it.

Old Testament laws, like the ones we have been discussing, flow from the dominant "Hebrew" perspective, under which a human being is essentially an animated (that is, breathed-into) body in which heart, kidneys, bowels, liver, inward parts, flesh, and bones all shape and determine character and emotions.[31] But in some later biblical writings, there are also traces of "Greek" influence, in which the human being is essentially an immortal soul that enters and informs a body prepared and ready for it.[32] In neither the Hebrew nor the Greek understanding is it intelligible to date personhood from conception. Hence, no biblical writer does so. Some scholars have suggested that the attention given to the conception of such key figures in the biblical narrative as Isaac, Samuel, John the Baptist, or Jesus implies a view that conception marks the true beginning of the human person in biblical terms.[33] It also has been suggested that the biblical description of pregnancy as "being with child" supports this view. But this is to push the evidence too far. It is only natural that, if one yearns for a child or looks forward to one who will inaugurate a new age, one will be interested in the fact of this conception as the necessary prolegomenon to the longed-for birth. Yet, the focus in all the accounts is entirely on the future birth and what the person will accomplish during his life.[34] None of this implies that personhood could be present from conception, and as we have seen, on no biblical understanding of personhood could such a view be founded.

The Tradition of the Church

Now although there do not seem to be any biblical grounds for regarding the fetus as a person, the situation might seem rather different when we turn to the tradition of the Church. For "all early Christian thinkers without exception rejected abortion,"[35] and according to Gerald Bonner, "until the 20th century, no serious Christian of any denomination would have attempted to defend abortion—if at all—except in the rarest and most exceptional circumstances."[36] Moreover, it is a plain fact of history that abortion and infanticide, which were a commonplace in the ancient Greco-Roman world, ceased to be so as Christian influence spread.[37] At first sight, therefore, there seems to be a strong case for claiming that those who wish to regard the fetus as a person and therefore oppose in-vitro research have Christian tradition on their side.

However, the issue is not so simple as this. For as the Church of England report on abortion points out, although Christians have insistently extended the protection of the law to the child in the womb, "at what point in its development the fetus became entitled to this protection was, from very early times, a matter of doubt."[38] The dominant view of the early Fathers was that, though abortion was always wrong, there was a radical difference between early and late abortion. Hence, no canonical penalties were incurred for an abortion carried out in the first 80 days of pregnancy,[39] and Augustine, Jerome and Thomas Aquinas all insisted that early abortion could not be classed as homicide.[40] According to Augustine, "there cannot be said to be a live soul in a body which lacks sensation, when it is not formed into flesh and so not yet endowed with sense."[41] In accordance with the medical beliefs of that time, the distinction between early and late abortion was characterized by talk of a difference between a "formed" and an "unformed" fetus or between an "animate" or "inanimate" one. The terms need not concern us, and we should use different expressions today; but they matter only as testimony to the deeply-felt conviction in the Christian tradition that there is a moral difference between the status of the fetus in the earliest stages of its development and in its later growth. What is important for our present purposes is that, for the first 1,900 years of the Christian tradition, a distinction was made between early and late abortion, and it is not possible to claim that the Fathers of the Church thought that the embryo was a human being from the moment of conception. They did not.[42]

The decisive change in the Roman Catholic attitude to the status of the early fetus stems from the proclamation of the dogma of the Immaculate Conception in 1854. In his statement, Pope Pius IX affirmed that "the Virgin Mary was, in the first instant of her conception, preserved untouched by any taint of original sin;"[43] but this is intelligible only if it can be supposed that Mary's personhood and moral sense could be thought of as already present "in the first instant of her conception." Consequently, Pius IX found it necessary to break with past teaching and insist that from the moment of conception a human being, with full status as a person, already exists. And so, in 1869, Pius IX dropped reference to an "ensouled fetus" in the grounds for excommunication for abortion, thus making, for the first time, early as well as late abortion a ground of excommunication.[44] This teaching was further explicated in the papal decrees of 1884, 1889 and 1902, which forbade direct termination of a pregnancy even in circumstances where, as in ectopic pregnancies, the result of non-intervention was the certain death of both mother and child.[45] It seems significant, however, that the Catholic conscience has not been willing to follow the implications of papal logic on this point, and a casuistry based on the doctrine of double effect now has been developed to circumvent the rigor of the papal pronouncements.[46] That in practice Catholic doctors find it morally impossible to treat the lives of fetus and mother as having equal significance is itself, I suggest, a ground for questioning the validity of the doctrine that asserts it.

If we then evaluate the elements in Christian tradition to which opponents of in-vitro research might appeal, we find that, apart from those who feel bound by the papal rulings of the last century, there is a relatively weak basis in the tradition for strong opposition to in-vitro research, even though a significant basis exists for opposing abortions carried out late in pregnancy. On the other hand, that personhood dates from conception has virtually no significant support in the tradition prior to the teaching of Pius IX.

Christian Reasoning

If neither the Bible nor Christian tradition offers much support for the dating of personhood from conception, what of Christian reasoning? By this I mean reasoning that operates within the framework of faith to present a coherent and intelligible account of the Christian vision of life. Some features of a Christian perspective include belief that God works through the life to create beings who can "feel after him and find him,"[47] entering into an eternal relationship with him that can triumph through death. It is pre-supposed that life has meaning and purpose and that the challenges and adversities of this life are, in some sense, necessary features of an existence that shapes the individual for his or her eternal destiny with God.[48]

The early Christians were worried that aborted fetuses, being unbaptized, would end up in Hell,[49] and their medieval successors speculated about the innocent, unbaptized living forever in the half-world of Limbo.[50] The mind boggles to think of the problems that such speculations would encounter today, when we know that in the ordinary course of nature, 70 percent of fertilized ova fail even to reach the stage of implantation.[51] According to Vatican II, salvation no longer depends on baptism,[52] and, according to Pope John Paul II, "every person, without exception, has been redeemed by Christ."[53] Yet, if belief in the universal salvific will of God[54] is joined to a belief that every single fertilized ovum is a human person, then Christians would have to postulate a heaven populated largely by unformed zygotes! Simply to state this implication is to indicate that Christian reason cannot acquiesce in so bizarre a conjunction of doctrines. Clearly, this problem could be circumvented by abandoning belief in a future life. But such a move would eradicate one of the central tenets of historical Christianity—one that seems essential to a coherent theology.[55]

Further, Christianity teaches that humanity is made in the image of God.[56] Traditionally, it has been supposed that it is in the capacity to reason that the likeness exists. However, "reason" in this context is not simply an intellectual matter, but is linked to a notion of the human person's having moral responsibility, spiritual awareness and aesthetic sensibility. Such qualities are not innate. They have to be developed, cultured and nourished throughout life. Hence, many Christian writers would have spoken of this world as "a vale of soul-making,"[57] expressing the view that what is most distinctive of personal character and individuality is shaped by the experiences of life through interaction with other human beings, through the tasks and duties of everyday life, and through communion with God. On this understanding of what it means to be a human being, it would simply be an absurdity to ascribe full possession of personhood to a newborn

60

baby, much less to a developing fetus, and still less to an embryo. Rather, personhood will not be something that can be categorically defined as present at any particular moment in time but will be described in terms of a continuum from almost nonexistence to the life of the mature adult and, if the Christian hope is realized, to fullest expression in the life of the world to come.

Hence, I suggest that, if a serious attempt is made to spell out a reasoned understanding of what Christian faith might mean today, it will be extremely hard to justify a dogmatic stance on the issue of in-vitro research.

Conclusion

I have tried to show that the current so-called Christian opposition to in-vitro fertilization research cannot legitimately find adequate justification by appeal to the Bible, church tradition or Christian reasoning. Hence, pressure groups have no right to invoke the moral weight of historic Christianity for their opinions. An alternative Christian response might recognize that, since the biological origin of each individual adult stretches back to the moment of his or her conception, it will be natural to feel a sense of concern about the appropriate use of human tissue and wish that embryonic research be adequately regulated and directed only to ends that enhance human welfare and fulfillment. It is important to note that almost all medical practitioners working in this area would be glad to support such a position.

NOTES

1. From the marriage service in the Anglican *Book of Common Prayer* (1662)
2. Interview in "Prospective nel Mondo," in D. Yallop, *In God's Name* (London: Guild, 1984), 200ff.
3. Letter from the President of the Royal College of Obstetricians and Gynecologists (Professor M. C. Macnaughton), *The Times*, November 29, 1984.
4. "Why Warnock Is Wrong," *The Times*, June 6, 1985.
5. In Britain, for example, both the major anti-abortion societies, Life and The Society for the Protection of Unborn Children are explicitly Christian in orientation, as are most books written against abortion.
6. General Synod Board for Social Responsibility, *Personal Origins* (London: Church Information Office, 1985); Free Church Federal Council/British Council of Churches, *Choices in Childlessness* (London: Free Church Federal Council, 1982).
7. Compare the article by Cardinal Hume cited in note 4, above, and note that the Catholic Bishops' Joint Committee on Bio-Ethical Issues also issued a strongly critical response to the Warnock Report in 1984, which claimed that "The destruction of human embryos...is the killing of human life." For an orthodox view, see M.O. Clement, "To Whom Does the Embryo Belong," in Robin Gill, *A Textbook of Christian Ethics* (Edinburgh: Clarke, 1985), 500.
8. Church Assembly Board for Social Responsibility, *Abortion: An Ethical Discussion* (London: Church Information Office, 1965). In the United States, the Episcopal church issued a policy statement on abortion that recognized the impossibility of defining the origins of life, and the Methodist church also adopted a liberal position (*The Times,* February 13, 1985).
9. Thirty percent of British wish the present law on abortion tightened, compared with 53 percent who wish it either to remain as it is or to be still further liberalized (*The Times,* February 2, 1980).
10. *Church Times,* July 22, 1983.
11. *The Times*, February 13, 1985.
12. Didaché 2:2. (There also may be biblical opposition to medicine in the condemnation of *pharmakeia* in Galatians 5:20, since although this is usually translated as a ban on sorcery, reference to any Greek dictionary will make clear that its primary meaning is "medicine, drug or remedy"; this is the meaning of "pharmacy" in every other context.)
13. For a polemical but well-documented account of all this, see A.D. White, *A History of the Warfare of Science with Theology,* vol. 2, (Cambridge: Harvard, 1985; London: Arco, 1955), 36ff.
14. Genesis 3:16.

15. A.D. White, *Warfare of Science with Theology*, vol. 2, 63.
16. See Paul Ramsey, *Fabricated Man* (New Haven: Yale, 1970), or O. O'Donovan, *Begotten or Made?* (Oxford: Clarendon, 1984).
17. Compare A.D. White, *Warfare of Science with Theology*, chapter 13.
18. Consider, for example, the widespread existence of clergy/doctors fellowship groups, or the membership of the Society for the Study of Religion and Medicine.
19. BBC Radio 4, "You and Yours," August 21, 1986.
20. Psalm 8.
21. Genesis 2:7.
22. P.D. Simmons, *Birth and Death: Bioethical Decision-making* (Philadelphia: Westminster, 1983), 86ff; and compare the Chief Rabbi's submission to the Warnock Committee cited in the General Synod Board for Social Responsibility, *Personal Origins*, 34.
23. Exodus 21:12.
24. Exodus 21:22.
25. Middle Assyrian laws, Tablet A:50, cited in J.B. Pritchard, *Ancient Near Eastern Texts Relating to the Old Testament* (Princeton: Princeton, 1950), 184.
26. Exodus 21:23.
27. Deuteronomy 22:21, Leviticus 21:9, Genesis 38:24.
28. P.D. Simmons, *Birth and Death*, 67.
29. Middle Assyrian laws, Tablet A: 53, cited in J.B. Pritchard, *Ancient Near Eastern Texts*, 185.
30. Clyde T. Francisco, *"Genesis,"* in *Broadman Bible Commentary*, vol. 1, 406, cited in P.D. Simmons, *Birth and Death*, 67.
31. W. Eichrodt, "The Components of Human Nature" in W. Eichrodt (ed.), *Theologie des Alten Testaments* (Stuttgart: Ehrenfried, trans., 1965), J.A. Baker, *Theology of the Old Testament* (London: SCM, 1967), chapter 16.
32. Wis. 8:20, 9:15; Ecclesiastes 11:5. And see discussion in P. Badham, "Soul," in J. Bowden, *New Dictionary of Christian Theology* (London: SCM, 1983).
33. Genesis 18:9-15, 21:1–2, 1 Samuel 1:1–20; Luke 1:5–45.
34. Genesis 17:19; 1 Samuel 1:11; Luke 1:13–17, 32-35.
35. C.S. Rodd, "Talking Points from Books," *The Expository Times*, vol. 97, (10) (July 1986), 290.
36. Gerald Bonner, "Abortion and Early Christian Thought," in J.H. Channer (ed.), *Abortion and the Sanctity of Life* (Exeter: Paternoster, 1985), 111.
37. W.E.H. Lecky, *History of European Morals*, vol. 2 (London: Longmans, Green, 1911), 20–34.
38. Church Assembly Board for Social Responsibility, *Abortion: An Ethical Discussion*, 17.
39. Church Assembly Board for Social Responsiblity, *Abortion*, 17.
40. General Synod Board for Social Responsibility, *Personal Origins*, 24–25.
41. Augustine on the Latin text, Exodus 21:22. Cited in General Synod Board

for Social Responsibility, *Personal Origins*, 24.

42. Gerald Bonner, "Abortion and Early Christian Thought" in J.H. Channer, *Abortion and the Sanctity of Life*, 113.

43. From the Bull *Ineffabilis Deus* of Pius IX, extract in Denzinger (1641) cited in H. Bettenson, *Documents of the Christian Church* (Oxford: Oxford, 1963) 381.

44. General Synod Board for Social Responsibility, *Personal Origins*, 25.

45. Church Assembly Board for Social Responsibility, *Abortion*, 27.

46. Church Assembly Board for Social Responsibility, *Abortion*, 27; R.F.R. Gardner, *Abortion* (Exeter: Paternoster, 1972), 99.

47. Acts 17:27.

48. Compare J. Hick, *Evil and the God of Love* (London: Macmillan, 1966).

49. W.E.H. Lecky, *The History of European Morals*, vol. 2, 23.

50. Jacques Le Goff, *La Naissance de Purgatoire* (Paris: Gaillimard, 1981), trans., A. Goldhammer, *The Birth of Purgatory* (London: Scholar, 1984), 220–221, 235–238.

51. *Lancet* 1 (January 26, 1980) 167.

52. C. Butler, *The Theology of Vatican II* (London: Darton, Longman & Todd, 1967), 112–113.

53. Cited in *Church Times*, May 23, 1986, from B. Meaking and J. Stott, *The Evangelical-Roman Catholic Dialogue on Mission* (Exeter: Paternoster, 1986).

54. K. Rahner, "Christianity and the Non-Christian Religions," in *Schriften Zur Theologie* (Einsiedeln: Verlagsanstalt Berzinger and Co., 1965) tran. K. H. Kruger, *Theological Investigations* (London: Darton, Longman & Todd, 1966), vol. 5, 118ff.

55. P. Badham, "In Search of Heaven," in *In Search of Christianity* (London: Weekend Television, 1986).

56. Genesis 1:27.

57. M.B. Forman (ed.), *The Letters of John Keats*, 4th ed. (London: Oxford, 1952), 333–335; cited in J. Hick, *Evil*, 295.

FOUR

CATHOLICISM And the VALUE Of HUMAN LIFE

Michael Coughlan

The Value of a Human Life

Steadfast Principle or Hyperbole?

"The Catholic Church once again stands fast on the priceless value of a human life." Thus ran the opening sentence of the editorial in a popular Catholic weekly in the U.K. following the issue of the Vatican instruction on embryo research and artificial procreation.[1] But such bold simplicity, however journalistically or rhetorically appealing, has to be treated with considerable caution. For instance, quite a natural interpretation of the claim that human life is priceless would be that such life may not be taken or sacrificed in any circumstances, and that it must be preserved whatever the costs (short, perhaps, of priceless costs). Yet, neither of these views has been adopted by the Church: capital punishment, killing in just war, or in self-defense, the foreseeable but unintended bringing about of deaths, the refusal to use "extraordinary means" to extend life—all of these have been, and still are, implicitly or explicitly condoned by the Church.

Are we to suppose that all of the aforementioned practices are compatible with the claim that human life is priceless, such that the proposed "natural interpretation" of this claim is in fact a misinterpretation? Let us consider, briefly, whether we could ever be justified in causing or allowing the loss of something held to be priceless. If anything could count as an adequate justification, surely it would have to be the defense, preservation, or securing of something which is itself deemed to be priceless. An instance of justification in this manner might be killing in self-defense. But killing in self-defense is treated by the Church as a special exception to the general rule that one may not kill in order to preserve life (e.g., one may not kill a fetal baby in order to save its mother's life), which is but one application of the inviolable "Pauline principle" that one may not do evil in order to secure a good.[2] This principle stands in stark opposition to the consequentialist principle, popularly stated as that the end may justify the means; more precisely, that actions are to be morally appraised purely in terms of their consequences—how those consequences are brought about is irrelevant (hence, killing a fetal baby may be justifiable if it will save the mother's life). Now whatever the declared position of the Church on the value of human life, it has consistently rejected consequentialism in favor of the "Pauline principle":

> ...it is never lawful, even for the gravest reasons, to do evil that good may come of it...even though the intention is to protect or promote the welfare of an individual, or a family or of society in general.[3]

But, given this position, what sense is there in speaking of "the priceless value of human life?" Human life, it appears, has its price: it may be, indeed *must be*, sacrificed if it can be defended only by evil means. If anything has priceless value from this perspective, it cannot be human life, or anything else which might be secured, enhanced, or promoted as a result of our actions. Such value must attach either to the actions themselves, or to some characteristic of them which is not determined by their consequences.

Lest this seem too short a way of dismissing the claim that the Church is committed to the pricelessness of human life, let us approach the issue from a different angle. It has to be admitted that many statements emanating from Rome appear at odds with this dismissal. In the document on embryo research it states: "From the moment of conception, the life of every human being is to be respected *in an absolute way...* (p. 11)." This is supported with a quote from the Holy See's Charter of Rights of the Family: "Human life must be *absolutely respected and protected* from the moment of conception" (p. 12—my italics in both quotes). These prescriptions cannot be taken to entail that one is under an absolute obligation to protect *any life* the fate of which lies in one's hands, for there are familiar moral dilemmas in which one is going to fail to protect *some* lives *whatever one chooses to do.* In these cases, it can be argued, provided that one does not sacrifice these lives as a means to protecting the others, one does not necessarily fail to show them absolute respect. But the Church has sanctioned, or condoned, the taking of human life in far less closely circumscribed situations than would fit these criteria. As Josef Fuchs, a respected Jesuit moral theologian, observes:

> ...the preservation or the taking of life are not, in themselves, an absolute value or an absolute evil, else it would not be permissible in any circumstances to kill or allow to die—and this is contrary to all tradition. Only a correct assessment of advantage, an assessment of the various values and evils implicit in an action (abstract or concrete) makes it possible to establish an absolute. In practice, moral theology has always applied this principle, for example to the question of what relevant values justify the killing of a man (e.g., capital punishment).[4]

Is it possible to take these considerations on board and still maintain a commitment to absolute respect for human life? Fuchs offers capital punishment as an example of justifiable killing, so let us give this issue a little attention. The defender of absolute respect for human life cannot justify capital punishment on teleological grounds, e.g., as an effective deterrent against murder or as protection for society, for this is to treat the life (or *death,* rather) of one individual as a tool for the benefit of others; as a mere means to an end. But it might seem that the institution of capital punishment is compatible with absolute respect for human life provided it is justified retributively, i.e., if executions are carried out only in the interests of justice. Indeed, it is often argued that absolute respect for human life *demands* the absolute punishment for murder. Whatever the degree of plausibility of this view on the theoretical level, a moment's reflection will reveal its inadequacy on the practical level. All human courts are fallible; therefore, to institute capital punishment is to risk taking innocent lives, i.e., to risk the grossest and utterly irreparable injustice. Such a risk, if it is justifiable at all, can be justified only teleologically. Therefore, the institution of capital punishment is incompatible with an *absolute* respect for human life.[5]

Numerous other examples of practices which have been traditionally accepted as permissible but which do not demand absolute respect for human life, or treating human life as priceless, could be cited (the justness of an action in a just war, for instance, and the placing of limits on the medical resources used to keep the critically ill alive). What, then, are we to make of these claims about the Church's teaching? We have to assume either that the Church has radically altered her position on a multitude of moral issues or that what we are being offered is hyperbole. The consequences of the former option would be radical, indeed, for a Church which lays claim to divinely guided teaching authority on moral matters. We may reasonably deduce, therefore, that this is not the correct assumption. But if it is hyperbole with which we are confronted—if Catholicism does not see human life as literally priceless, or literally requiring absolute respect—what value or respect does it command, and how is this grounded?

Divine Law and Natural Law

Rather than trying to answer this last question by cleaving through the hyperbolic prose, it might be more profitable to start with first principles. For Catholicism, as for Christianity in general and, indeed, any monotheistic religion, ultimate value must surely lie in the Deity itself, and ultimate obligation in doing the will of the Deity. For any religion with its roots in Judaism, the consequences of this commitment are most vividly illustrated by Abraham's experience in being divinely commanded to sacrifice his son, Isaac.[6] In this passage, it is made expressly clear that all human values must be yielded before the will of God. Much Protestant thinking has deduced from this that guidance in ethical issues is a matter of direct revelation or intuition of the

68

divine will in each particular situation; that there are no universally valid rules such as that one may not take an innocent human life. Catholic thought, on the other hand, has insisted that the divine will is ordinarily revealed to us *indirectly*, either authoritatively, through the scriptures and the teaching of the Church, or rationally, through the perceptible order of nature which is itself an expression of the divine will. That which is revealed to us authoritatively is referred to as the Divine Law; that which is revealed to us rationally is the Natural Law.

Divine Law never conflicts with Natural Law (for how could the divine will be in conflict with itself?), but it both overlaps Natural Law, frequently confirming its precepts, and extends beyond it, e.g., in prescribing that the Sabbath be kept holy. As the Divine Law includes the Natural Law, the Church lays claim to the position of authoritative interpreter of the latter, despite its being rationally accessible. The argument is that, given the fallibility of human reason and the susceptibility of human judgment to be swayed by sinfulness, an unerring authority on the moral law is indispensable if we are to have sure knowledge of the divine will for us. Nonetheless, the Church does teach that neither direct revelation nor its teaching authority is *essentially* required for a knowledge of Natural Law, and, consequently, Natural Law constitutes the basic moral law for all humankind.

What do we learn from Natural Law about the value of human life? Both Catholic moral theology and Church teaching have been less than explicit about this. One critical commentator remarks:

> ...I should like to point out a fact about (Catholic) clerical education which may have something to do with the defects of the argument from nature. In seminaries and clerical universities, it seems to be nobody's job to expound the argument. The course in moral philosophy does not include it, and the course in moral theology mentions it only as something presumed to be already familiar.[7]

This writer was directly concerned with the argument from Natural Law against contraceptive practices, but the point might be given a general application. Indeed, Natural Law ethics has been more explicitly formulated in relation to sexual practices than in relation to any other moral sphere. When Pope Paul VI endorsed the "Pauline principle" (p. 2, above), the evil he had in mind was the "intrinsic wrong" of "sexual intercourse which is deliberately contraceptive." The intrinsic wrongfulness of this practice resides in its direct conflict with the Natural Law, which prescribes the unitive and procreative functions of sexual intercourse must not be separated:

> The reason is that the marriage act, because of its fundamental structure, while uniting husband and wife in the closest intimacy, actualizes their capacity to generate new life—and this as a result of laws written into the actual nature of man and woman.[8]

From this text we may infer something concerning the characteristics of Natural Law argumentation, at least as presented by the Church's teaching authority. It is the "fundamental structure" of the act which is crucial, and which must be *absolutely* respected.[9] Any interference with, or departure from, this fundamental structure cannot be justified, even for the most weighty considerations. Hence, deliberately contraceptive sexual intercourse, masturbation, sodomy, bestiality, etc., can all be morally ruled out without any inquiry into the circumstances of their practice: *nothing* outside of the structure of the act itself is relevant. In this, these prohibitions differ radically from the prohibition, if it is one, against killing human beings. Whether an act is an act of masturbation or sodomy can be specified in nonmoral terms, and the moral judgment, on the Natural Law argument, is wholly implicit in that specification. Whether an act is an act of killing is equally specifiable in nonmoral terms, but the moral judgment cannot, or at least cannot in the view of the Church, be deduced from that specification: the moral setting of the killing has to be taken into consideration.[10] It might seem that all we need to secure a comparable methodology of evaluation in the killing case is to specify the act more precisely, e.g., what is intrinsically wrong is the *direct* killing of *innocent* human life. But this will not do, for whether the killing is "direct" or the victim is "innocent" cannot be determined from the "fundamental structure" of the act alone.

This treatment of the physical structure of actions as crucial in determining their moral quality has long been criticized by Protestant moral theologians and is now increasingly shunned by their Catholic counterparts. As one of the latter, significantly one currently under a cloud of Church disapprobation, Charles Curran, remarks: "...there exists a definite chasm between the way many moral theologians do moral theology and the approach employed in the official teaching of the hierarchical magisterium."[11] But the consequence of this is not that we get from the moral theologians more clarity on the issue of when killing is unjustifiable, but rather that the kind of contextual reasoning brought to bear in deciding this issue is also brought to bear on issues in sexual practice.

There is, however, a straightforward argument in Natural Law ethics for a *prima facie* obligation (i.e., an obligation which is binding, all else being equal, but one which may be overridden by other obligations in certain circumstances) to respect or promote human life. The first principle of Natural Law is that good is to be done and promoted and evil avoided. Human life, in itself, is taken to do something good. Therefore, human life is to be promoted. But this argument, as so far stated, is no stronger than analogous arguments for canine life, or bovine life, or any other form of life. (Incidentally, it has been observed that if the Natural Law arguments against interference in the sexual order are sound, then they are equally telling against, e.g., sterilization or artificial insemination of livestock.[12]) Although one can reinforce the human case by pointing to the greater good inherent in human life, i.e., that it includes the values of conscious or sensitive life, but also transcends them with the value of self- conscious, rational life; nevertheless, the Natural Law argument yields a *prima facie* case against killing nonhuman life which the Church, as interpreter of the Natural Law, has not been at pains to teach. On the contrary, the idea of Albert Schweitzer that *all* life demands reverence comes in for some sharp criticism by two of the more orthodox and highly influential Catholic moral theologians, John Ford and Gerald Kelly:

> In a word, Dr. Schweitzer's thesis on reverence for life is simply sugar-coated moral poison. He wishes to avoid destroying any life, even the lowest; but he sadly realizes that some such destruction is "necessary." And when it is "necessary," it is permitted. The logical conclusion of this supposedly magnificent thesis...is that even innocent human life may be directly destroyed when this is "necessary."[13]

That which induces Catholic moral theologians and the church to raise the value of human life (and the values inherent in human sexuality) onto a plane wholly distinct from that of all other life is surely not something implicit in the natural order, but theological doctrine. It is now timely to complete the quotation cited earlier from the *Instruction* on embryo research:

> From the moment of conception, the life of every human being is to be respected in an absolute way because man is the only creature on earth that God has "wished for himself" and the spiritual soul of each is "immediately created" by God; his whole being bears the image of the Creator. Human life is sacred because from its beginning it involves "the creative action of God" and it remains forever in a special relationship with the Creator, who is its sole end. God alone is the Lord of life from its beginning until its end; no one can, in any circumstance, claim for himself the right to destroy directly an innocent human being.[14]

The authoritativeness of this statement is underlined by no less than seven references in the footnotes, including reference to four popes and the documents of the Second Vatican Council.

Is this statement intended to be understood as an interpretation of the Natural Law or as an exposition of Divine Law which is supplementary to the Natural Law? Some moral theologians would prefer that this distinction were dropped entirely,[15] but, although that desire may be understandable from a Catholic point of view, others may wish to know, and it is intelligible to ask, whether this teaching is based wholly on special revelation or whether it is meant to be evident through rational investigation of the natural order. An unambiguous answer was provided by Pope Paul VI:

> The question of the birth of children, like every other question which touches human life, is too large to be resolved by limited criteria, such as are provided by biology, psychology, demography or sociology. It is the whole man and the whole complex of his responsibilities that must be considered, *not only what is natural and limited to this earth, but also what is supernatural and eternal.*[16] (My italics.)

Pope Pius XII had made effectively the same point in discussing the theological-cum-moral significance of evolutionary theory.[17] Thus, despite repeated appeals to Natural Law as a basis for its moral teachings, this Law, understood as the order in nature which is accessible to human reason, is admitted to be an insufficient basis for the Catholic evaluation of human life. It is not the human being's place *within* the natural order, but rather her or his *relationship with the divine* which constitutes the only adequate basis for the Catholic view.

"From the Moment of Conception…"

The Church's view, therefore, is that it is God's will that human beings should have a unique place in the moral order, and this is expressed in particular by God's "immediate creation" of their spiritual souls. The notion of "immediate creation" of the soul has a long tradition in Catholic theology and recurs frequently in Papal and Roman documents, including, as seen above, the recent *Instruction* on embryo research. It does *not* mean that the soul is created immediately upon conception, but rather that its creation is a direct act of God and not something which God does through the mediation of the natural order. The soul, being immaterial and spiritual, cannot be a product of biological forces. It is this spiritual soul which sets humankind apart from all other kinds of being: it is that which makes it possible for us to remain "forever in a special relationship with the Creator."[18]

An important issue for the moral standing of the conceptus or of the embryo will be whether it has been invested with a spiritual soul. The authors of the *Instruction* on embryo research, while recognizing that: "The Magisterium has not expressly committed itself to an affirmation of a philosophical nature…,"[19] seem intent on nudging us firmly in that direction. Although the *Instruction* admits that "Physical life, with which the course of human life in the world begins, certainly does not itself contain the whole of a person's value…," it goes on to state that:

> The inviolability of the innocent human being's right to life "from the moment of conception until death" is a sign and requirement of the very inviolability of the person to whom the Creator has given the gift of life.[20]

How can the inviolability of the person *require* inviolability from the moment of conception unless it is assumed that there exists a person from that moment? It has to be understood here that "person" in the Catholic tradition has been understood in the sense first given to it by Boethius, viz., an individual substance of a rational nature. The rational nature is the nature of the spiritual soul, that which transcends animal nature and gives the individual the special relationship with God. The *Instruction,* along with much Catholic thinking on this issue, trades on the ambiguity between the notion of a person and that a human being, as it also trades on the ambiguity between "human life" and "life of a human being." The Second Vatican Council decreed that "from the moment of its conception, (human) life must be guarded with the greatest care"[21] and, as already noted, the *Instruction* refers to the statement in the Holy See's *Chapter of the Rights of the Family* that "human life must be absolutely respected and protected from the moment of conception." In the *Instruction,* however, the formula, already quoted on two occasions, is: "From the moment of conception, the life of every human being is to be respected in an absolute way...." It is noteworthy that the Second Vatican Council deliberated at length on the form of expression required in this context, and the formula incorporated into its documents was specifically selected so that the question of the point of ensoulment was not touched upon.[22] It is scarcely questionable that there is human life at this stage, but to speak of the life of *a human being* comes at least very close to begging this issue.

The authors of the *Instruction* also offer a staged argument in favor of the view that a person exists from the moment of conception, part of which is drawn from an earlier document issued by the same body.[23] In summary, the argument runs as follows: As the life of the fertilized ovum is neither the life of the father nor that of the mother, it is a *new* life. This new life is a *human* life, for it could not be made human if it were not human already. Third, from the first instant the biological identity of the new human *individual* is already constituted. And finally, it is asked rhetorically, what could this new human individual be but a human person?

As this argument is clearly intended as a contribution to the philosophical debate, a philosophical response would not be inappropriate. While a great deal could be said, space permits only an outline of some objections the argument needs to meet:

a) It is undeniable that the life of the *fertilized* ovum is a new life in the sense that it is a life which is neither that of the father alone nor that of the mother alone. Yet, it is in a sense, and in a very precious sense to the parents, a life of *both* the father and the mother: if its life derived in no way from theirs, that would radically alter their relationship to it. More profoundly significant, perhaps, is the possibility of embryonic life which *is derived from the father or the mother alone.* Catholic moral theology is eventually going to have to come to terms with parthenogenetic reproduction. Although the *Instruction* does mention attempts to obtain human beings through parthenogenesis in order to condemn the practice,[24] it leaves unanswered the question of the implications of such possibilities for the argument under consideration.

b) One would hardly wish to deny that the life of the conceptus is human life, but unless other questions are being begged, all that can mean here is that it is constituted of living human cells. In other words, the remark's significance is biological and nothing more. The individual gametes, sperm and ova, before union in fertilization, are also human life in this sense. If it is objected that without union they do not have the biological dynamism of growth or cleavage, then once again this overlooks the possibilities raised by parthenogenesis. Incidentally, the implication in the argument that that which is not human could never become human, which must surely be intended here in the biological sense, appears to raise an insuperable difficulty for the theory of evolution (which is not consonant with the Church's outlook on this theory).

c) But it is the notions of identity and individuality through the fertilization to implantation period which pose the greatest philosophical difficulties, and these difficulties are not, as the *Instruction* suggests, alleviated by recent scientific findings, but rather aggravated by them. We start with an individual cell with a unique genetic combination. But the difficulties of describing that cell as an individual human being are manifold. Firstly, it begins to multiply by division or cleavage. The cell group at this stage may split into two units, leading to the development of identical twins (the genetic combination is then no longer unique). This poses a difficulty for the idea of ensoulment at conception, a difficulty with which Catholic thinkers have sought to meet by postulating the infusion of a second soul at the point of division. But this solution creates a number of problems of its own. If this is what happens, then, strictly speaking, the second individual is not the offspring of the parents, but a product of the first individual; we would have a single parent family in the womb! In any case, there seem to be no grounds for distinguishing one of the emerging twins as the primary and the other as the secondary, the process being a symmetrical division of the cell group or mass.

Further, while it is correct to say that from the early embryo, all else being satisfactory, at least one unique individual will develop. That does not entail that at least one unique individual is already present in the early embryo, or even that it makes sense to think that there might be. We have to look at what kind of entity the embryo is, and specifically, at whether the individuality of the individuals which develop from it is determined intrinsically, i.e., does their uniqueness have its basis in features which are internal to the embryo and already present from the moment of conception? We shall look at this question in a moment. Before that, it needs to be pointed out that the second-soul-creation response to the problem of identical twinning generates an added difficulty for itself when the phenomenon of recombination is considered, i.e., it is possible for an embryo which had split into twin units to recombine into a single unit. Whether this happens naturally in human embryos has been questioned,[24a] but there are no reasons for ruling it out *a priori*—medically it is conceivable, if unlikely. An account of soul acquisition, which is not prone to fall at the next advance in knowledge of the development of the embryo, must be able to cope with this possibility. But if recombination occurs, nothing has perished, i.e., no human tissue has perished. What then has happened to the second soul? It looks as though we have had a death without a body, and apart from any other considerations, theological problems arise in connection with the doctrine of the resurrection of the body. An attempted solution might be to hold that God foresees (or that He predetermines) the recombination and does not, therefore, infuse the briefly independent cell group with a soul. But this suggests a connection between body and soul or a more highly contingent order than the Catholic Church tradition, at least since the time of Thomas Aquinas, has been prepared to admit.

The occurrence of identical twins has no apparent genetic determinant. Rather, it seems to be the result of causal factors extraneous to the embryonic cells themselves. In fact, every healthy embryo could generate at least four identical human beings, given the appropriate cultivation of the embryonic cells, for, at least up to the four-cell stage, each cell is "toti-potential," i.e., capable of separate development into a full human body. Now if it is supposed that the original toti-potential cell is a unique individual such that it might be possessed of a soul, is it to be supposed that the four-cell embryo is this same unique individual or is each of the four toti-potential cells a unique individual by itself, one identical with the original and three new arrivals? I doubt if the latter would be contended, but if it were, it would have to face a multiplication of the problems mentioned in connection with the recombination of identical twins. If this is *not* supposed to be the case, i.e., if it is supposed that there is still only one unique individual, then we have some puzzling moral issues arising. What, e.g., has been done by the gynecologist who extracts one of the four toti-potential cells from the embryo because it can be seen to be malformed, leaving the remainder to develop into a normal fetus, and destroying the extracted cell? On the supposition that each toti-potential cell at this stage is not a unique individual, he cannot have destroyed a unique individual—he simply disposed of some damaged tissue for the benefit of the embryonic individual which survives. Yet, what he destroys has no less potential for development as a unique individual than the original toti-potential cell; had it been placed in the shell of an emptied unfertilized ovum which was then implanted in a womb, it could have grown into a fully-fledged fetus.

The possibility of the splitting of the cell group, leading to the formation of identical twins, remains until implantation, i.e., about two weeks after fertilization of the embryo. Before that time, the foregoing observations indicated the inappropriateness of speaking of the cell mass as an individual human being. Further, as leading Catholic moral theologian Bernard Häring remarks: "In our philosophical tradition it is a common presupposition that only a human life possessing irreversible individuality can be a person."[25] Indeed, it might be added, irreversibly individual human life is but a minimal requirement for being a person: the quality of that life has to be appropriate, too. This point has a long tradition in Catholic philosophical psychology. To quote from some of the comparatively more recent literature (bearing in mind that becoming a person is interpreted as becoming ensouled):

> *a)* Cardinal Mercier, in 1916, noting the suggestion that ensoulment is the moment of conception, wrote:

...it is...much more probable that the soul is created during the course of embryonic life.... The organic development of the body is a gradual process;...Life first unfolds itself as the result of an organic principle similar to that in plants; next, sensibility appears in virtue of an animal form...; until finally the embryo has attained all the dispositions requisite for its being vivified by a rational soul.[26]

> *b)* Karl Rahner, acclaimed the greatest Catholic theologian of this century, finds an analogy between the evolutionary process and embryo development:

In both cases a not yet human biological organism develops towards a condition in which the coming into existence of a spiritual soul has its sufficient biological substratum.[27]

This approach to the issue of ensoulment, along the Natural Law ethical theory, is part of the Catholic intellectual heritage from Thomas Aquinas. Thomas' notion, derived from Aristotle, of human development as progression through a sequence of life forms, from the vegetative, through the sensitive/motive, to the rational/spiritual, with each stage incorporating rather than supplanting the former, far from being outdated, is remarkably consonant with current scientific knowledge. If rationally accessible knowledge of the natural order, through science and philosophy, is to count for anything, it must be counted, emphatically and enduringly, as pointing *away* from the conclusion that it makes sense to speak of ensoulment, or of the existence of a person, from the moment of conception.

Note that even if the Church were to accept this conclusion, it would not materially alter its moral stand on the inviolability of the embryo. There would still remain the teaching that, by Natural Law, the human generative process is sacrosanct, i.e., the teaching on which the prohibition of contraception is based, also has application to the generative process *after* conception. However, in this situation the *nature* of the objection to embryo research and in-vitro fertilization techniques would be very different from that which is suggested by the emotive closing quotation of the *Instruction*: "What you do to one of the least of my brethren, you do unto me." (Matthew 25:40).

NOTES

1. *The Universe*, No. 6562, 13th March 1987. The instruction referred to is the document: *Instruction on Respect for Human Life in its Origin and on the Dignity of Procreation*, issued by the Congregation for the Doctrine of the Faith (London: Catholic Truth Society, 1987), (hereafter: *Instruction*).
2. *Epistle of St. Paul to the Romans* 3:8 and 6:1f.
3. *Encyclical Letter of Pope Paul VI: Humanae Vitae* (London: Catholic Truth Society, 1968), (hereafter *Humanae Vitae*, $14).
4. Josef Fuchs, *Human Values and Christian Morality* (Dublin: Gill and Mac-Millan, Dublin 1970), 198n.
5. If it should be retorted that its abolition, too, would be incompatible with absolute respect for human life, then that may be admitted. The lesson is that absolute respect for human life is something which we are not in a position to exercise.
6. Genesis 22:1–18.
7. G. Egner, *Birth Regulation and Catholic Belief: A Study in Problems and Possibilities* (London and Melbourne: 1966), 70n.
8. Pope Paul VI, *Humanae Vitae*, $12.
9. *Ibid.*, $11.
10. For an extended treatment of this point, see Egner, *op. cit.*.
11. Charles E. Curran, *Transition and Tradition in Moral Theology* (Notre Dame: University of Notre Dame Press, 1979), 18.
12. See Egner, 44f.
13. John C. Ford, and Gerald Kelly, *Contemporary Moral Theology*, vol. 1, (Cork: Mercier Press, 1958), 9.
14. *Instruction*, 11.
15. E.g., Fuchs, *op. cit.*, 14.
16. Pope Paul VI: *Humanae Vitae*, $7.

17. In the encyclical *Humani Generis,* published in 1950.
18. *Instruction,* 11. Cf. *Pastoral Constitution on the Church in the Modern World,* art. 24 in *The Documents of Vatican II,* W.M. Abbott ed. (London and Dublin: Chapman, 1966), (hereafter: *The Church Today*).
19. *Instruction,* 13.
20. *Ibid.,* 10.
21. *The Church Today,* Art. 51.
22. See B. Häring, *Medical Ethics* (Slough: St. Paul Publications, 1974), 76.
23. Congregation for the Doctrine of the Faith, *Declaration on Procured Abortion,* 1974: see *Instruction,* 13. For a philosophical defense of similar arguments by a Catholic philosopher, see Germain Grisez, *Abortion: The Myths, the Realities and the Arguments* (New York: Corpus, 1970).
24. *Instruction,* 19.
25. T.W. Hilgers, "Human Reproduction: Three Issues for the Moral Theologian," *Theological Studies* 38 (1977), 136–152.
26. Häring, *op. cit.,* 80.
27. Mercier *et al., A Manual of Modern Scholastic Philosophy,* trans. by T.L. Parker and S.A. Parker, vol. 1 (London: Kegan Paul, 1916), 318.
28. K. Rahner, *Hominisation: The Evolutionary Origin of Man as a Theological Problem,* W.T. O'Hara (translator), (London: Burns and Oates, 1965).

FIVE

BIRTH CONTROL And the VALUE Of HUMAN LIFE

Shigemi Kono

Rise of the Population Concern

Since Thomas Robert Malthus published his celebrated *Essay on the Principle of Population*,[1] the threat of population growth has become the concern of social scientists, government administrators and political leaders alike in both the developed and developing countries. However, the question of population has been subdued for more than 100 years, while the Western world underwent the historically unprecedented and profound economic and industrial transformation called "the industrial revolution," accompanying technological innovations in the fields of manufacturing, agriculture, transportation and communication. During the period of the industrial revolution, food production increased tremendously and, in spite of the substantial population growth which followed, the standard of living in Europe and Northern America (U.S.A. and Canada) increased on an unprecedented scale. Accordingly, the population issue had been regarded as "solved," and, furthermore, population growth had been considered not only no menace to the nation, but also an essentially positive element for thrusting economic development and increase in the nation's well-being.

Nevertheless, the ghost of Malthus has not disappeared completely from the world. It started haunting again in the Third World after World War II, taking a different guise. Immediately after that war, the Third World consisting of Asia, Latin America, Africa and Oceania, excluding Australia and New Zealand, experienced spectacular population increases. The increases were unprecedentedly large in the number and relative intensity (in terms of growth rate). In 1950, the world population was 2.5 billion. In 1960, it became 3 billion, in 1975, it increased to 4.1 billion, and in 1987, it reached 5 billion. During the 19th century, the world population had grown at an annual average rate of only 0.5 percent. During 1900–1950, the annual average rate of growth increased to a modest rate of 0.8 percent. But in 1950–1955 the rate of growth of the world population jumped to 1.8 percent and in 1965–1970 it increased to an unprecedented rate of 2.0 percent per annum. Although in the most recent 10 years of 1975–1985 the rate has been reduced to 1.7 percent, each year the population approximating that of the country of Mexico, or 77 million, has been added to the world population. According to the most authoritative United Nations population projections made in 1985, the world population would reach 6.1 billion by the year 2000, 8.2 billion by 2025, and 10.1 billion by 2100. It is very important to note that during the 35 years between 1950 and 1985, the population growth of the Third World countries accounted for 85 percent of the world population growth. In 1950, the percentage share of the Third World was 67 percent or two-thirds of the world population. In 1985, it has increased to 75.7 percent or three-quarters. In the year 2025, it will become 83 percent or five-sixths. As far as population numbers are concerned, the 21st century will be predominantly a century for the Third World, particularly for Africa and South Asia. On the other hand, East Asia and Latin America have deceleration of population growth.

The rapid population growth in the developing countries after the termination of World War II has been called the "population explosion," or the big bang of the population bomb. The rapidity and enormity of this population explosion are simply historically unprecedented. But, why had such a phenomena appeared in the Third World after the war? Was this because of the substantial gains which had taken place in the Third World countries in the area of food production and enhancement of living standards accompanying gains in nutritional and calorific intake? The answer is a very qualified yes, but that was certainly not the main reason. Some developing countries might have experienced an expansion in food production and improvement in the standard of living, but many did not gain much either in food production or in standard of living. The population growth in the Third World took place by a reduction of mortality without any accompanying reduction in fertility. The main reason was the mortality decline attributable to the import to the Third World of the essential outcomes of the developments in the medical sciences and in technology in the developed countries of Northern America and Europe immediately after the war, and particularly the development of antibiotics, insecticides and other public health measures, inoculation and immunization, purification and sterilization of drinking water and milk, etc. In a country like Sri Lanka (formerly Ceylon), killing mosquitoes by spraying DDT, cleaning up ditches, drying out water ponds and swamps had resulted in reducing malaria casualities on a big scale, and this led to a tremendous reduction in mortality. Between the periods 1936–1946 and 1950–1952, the crude death rate of Ceylon declined from 21 to 12 per 1,000 population.

To summarize, the enormous reduction in mortality in the Third World was made by the implantation of Western medical sciences and public health technology and did not necessarily accompany substantial improvement in the standard of living or in nutritional or calorific conditions. It is important that in the Third World countries the reduction in mortality occurred mostly alone, without concurrence of fertility reduction. In Europe and Northern America, on the other hand, fertility started declining with a time lag of a few decades after mortality had started falling in the late 18th century or early 19th century. As a general historical trend in the demographic transition, mortality decline is normally followed by fertility decline. We shall explain the reasons for this later.

Population growth is the balance between births and deaths, if we do not consider migration. Obviously, the recent population explosion in the developing countries means that mortality has declined substantially, but fertility has not equally declined. It should be noted, however, that in very recent years, as already mentioned, the rate of population growth for the developing countries has been declining. In 1965–1970 the rate of population growth for the developing countries was 2.5 percent; in 1970–1975 it declined to 2.4 percent and in 1975–1980 it was further reduced to 2.1 percent. In the latest quinquennium of 1980–1985, the same rate has been 2.0 percent. In spite of the fact that mortality has continuously and appreciably been curtailed at the same time, the reduction in population growth rate means that there has been a notable decline in fertility or birth rate in the past two decades. The demographic statistics amassed by the United Nations Population Division tell us that the recent decline of fertility in China has played a big role in bringing down the birth rate of the developing countries as a whole, accounting for its 55 percent. This can be imputed predominantly to the bold planning and successful implementation of the one-child population policy there.

The next question will be concerned with the conditions for fertility decline in the Third World which is necessarily related to birth control and its underlying philosophy, or "family planning" in more current usage. We shall first review the reasons why fertility has declined in both the developed (including Japan, which is the sole industrialized country outside countries of European descent and culture) and developing countries; then we shall make assessments of the role of family planning played in the reduction in both developed and developing countries; and, finally, we shall discuss some ethical questions relating to birth control and population in a more widely conceived frame of reference.

Conditions for Fertility Decline

Table 5-1 indicated the trends of fertility in the world by the more developed and less developed regions and by eight major areas, namely Africa, Latin America, Northern America, East Asia, South Asia, Europe, Oceania and the U.S.S.R. according to

TABLE 5-1

Trends of World Population Growth by the More Developed and Less Developed Regions and by Major Areas

Regions	Crude Birth Rate				Total Fertility Rate			
	1950-1955	1960-1965	1970-1975	1980-1985	1950-1955	1960-1965	1970-1975	1980-1985
World	37.3	35.3	31.6	27.1	4.94	4.95	4.44	3.52
More Developed	22.7	20.3	17.0	15.5	2.80	2.66	2.1	1.97
Less Developed	44.4	41.9	37.2	31.0	6.12	6.07	5.40	4.06
Africa	48.3	48.2	46.8	45.9	6.47	6.59	6.50	6.34
America	33.8	32.5	27.1	25.3	4.63	4.69	3.63	3.14
Latin America	42.5	41.0	35.4	31.6	5.86	5.94	5.01	4.09
Northern America	25.1	22.8	16.5	15.9	3.43	3.31	19.5	1.83
Asia	42.7	39.5	34.9	27.2	5.87	5.72	5.06	3.54
East Asia	40.8	35.5	29.4	18.8	5.68	5.32	4.37	2.34
South Asia	44.6	43.2	39.8	34.1	6.04	6.08	5.67	4.59
Europe	19.8	18.7	16.1	13.9	2.56	2.59	2.16	1.88
Oceania	27.6	26.7	25.0	20.7	3.78	3.89	3.15	2.65
U.S.S.R.	26.3	22.3	17.8	19.0	2.82	2.54	2.44	2.35

Note: Both crude death rate and total fertility rate are the annual average for five years.

Source: United Nations, *World Population Prospects: Estimates and Projections as Assessed in 1984*, 1986. (Made available in the form of computer printout).

the United Nations classification. Two measures of fertility are used: one is crude birth rate and the other total fertility rate. Crude birth rate is the simplest indicator of fertility, which is obtained by dividing the number of births by the mid-period or the mean population in the period concerned. This is a useful indicator since the balance between this and the corresponding crude death rate signifies the rate of natural increase, but its drawback is that it does not take into account difference in population composition: if the population is young and particularly if it has a high proportion of females aged 20–29, as in the Philippines, then the population tends to have a higher birth rate. On the other hand, in the case of an aged population, like Sweden, where the female population aged 20–29 is relatively low, the crude birth rate tends to be lower even though the average number of children that a couple bears is the same as in the Philippines. In contrast to crude birth rate, total fertility rate does not have this bias created by age composition. It is calculated by summing up all the age-specific birth rates, each of which is obtained by dividing the number of births occurring to a female population of a particular age x by the corresponding female population aged x. In other words, the total fertility rate is the standardized birth rate (standardized by age in order not to have the effect of different age composition), provided that the weight of population for each age is a unity, that is one.

So much for the explanation of the two measures of fertility. Let us now look at Table 5-1. The first observation to make is the marked contrast in the level of fertility between the more developed and less developed regions. In 1950–1955, the crude birth rate for the more developed regions was 22.7, while that for the less developed was at 44.4, being almost twice as high a rate as for the more developed. In 1980–1985, although both the regions underwent considerable decreases from 1950–1955 to 1980–1985, their relative positions were the same in relation to each other. The less developed regions show twice as high a rate as the more developed ones. If we turn to the total fertility rate, the contrast is even more prominent. In 1950–1955 the total fertility rate for the less developed is more than twice as high as that for the more developed. In 1980–1985, their relative positions to each other remain much the same; fertility has declined substantially in the less developed regions, but a substantial decline also has taken place in the more developed regions.

Looking into the differences in major geographical areas, contrasts are even more conspicuous. In terms of total fertility rate, in 1980–1985 Africa indicates 6.34, whereas Northern America, comprising mostly the United States of America and Canada, signifies only 1.83. By the way, in terms of total fertility rate, the level of 2.1 is the cutting-off point in terms of net replacement of population in the next generation for the developed countries where mortality is low and life expectancy is high. If the rate is below 2.1, the population will decline eventually if not in the immediate future. Since there are some demographic inertia involving people already born, the population may grow even when the total fertility rate is below 2.1. If the rate is well above 2.1 the population will continuously increase. It depends to some extent on the level of mortality as was already implied. If mortality is high and the life expectancy is high in the developing countries, then the total fertility rate of 2.5 or 2.6 is the cutting-off point for the net replacement level. It is also noted that among the four major areas of less developed countries, namely Africa, Latin America, East Asia and South Asia, there are considerable variations in the level of fertility. If we take total fertility rate, we note that East Asia shows the most rapid decline between 1950–1955 and 1980–1985, being reduced to less than a half of the original level of 1950–1955. On the other hand, in Africa, the fertility rate has been virtually the same. Latin America and South Asia are in between and each exhibits a moderate extent of decline. This means that the less developed regions or the Third World countries are not uniform in this respect but show a considerable level of diversity.

At any rate, the important question remains as to why the less developed regions tend to show a higher fertility, while the more developed regions are prone to express a lower fertility. Common sense dictates that this is utterly upside down. Because they are rich in per capita income and, hence, in economic capability, the more developed countries should have had and could have had a higher birth rate, whereas being poor in per capita income and, hence, in economic capacity, the less developed should have had a lower fertility. But the reality is completely the reverse of this and one may be forced to think that there must be some good but complicated reasons to explain why the more developed have a lower fertility and the less developed have a higher fertility.

The trend to low fertility among the more developed countries dates back to the industrial revolution, when the standard of living was enhanced by the increase in manufacturing and agricultural productivity and when the processes of urbanization, secularization and literacy proceeded. The combined forces of the increase in standard of living, urbanization, secularization and the spread of education particularly to women, first reduced mortality and at the same time gave people the idea of practicing fertility control. Reduction in mortality, which particularly cut down infant and child mortality, generated some overpopulation in each household and community, thus creating a population problem there. But the very philosophical thinking which promoted mortality decline tended to push down fertility also. We may refer to a kind of rational way of thinking evolved in urban-industrial settings, in consonance with the desire for providing decent, clean and orderly life and in consonance with a philosophy that individual behavior and action remains in the domain of human choice. Some people already knew some premodern techniques of contraception, such as coitus interruptus, douching, or the use of rudimentary condoms and intrauterine contraceptive devices, though these methods had not been well disseminated among the people. Still, there existed taboos and inhibitions which regarded anything related to sex as vulgar and profane. It is argued that in the process of secularization and urbanization, people would have come to realize that controlling their fertility was not against the prevailing religious belief and folkways and mores.

Again, there are many reasons why fertility is high in the developing countries. First of all, the people there do not have access to the idea that family planning can generally be accepted or is a good thing for the society where they live; and besides, the people do not have access to the knowledge and know-how of methods of controlling fertility. According to Himes, human beings have been practicing contraception even from the very ancient time, but the point is that the knowledge of how to do it has not been made available to the general public.[2]

Another dimension of thought relates to the utility and cost of raising children in the rural and agricultural setting. In the developing countries, where agriculture is a predominant form of economic activity, the value of children is very high. First of all, children are useful as a labor force at the time of planting seeds and harvesting crops. Second, in the agrarian societies of developing countries, people lack social security systems so that when parents get aged, children, particularly male children, are supposed to be the main source of social security for the parents. After all, when parents get aged and incapacitated or bedridden, incapable of economic activities, sons are supposed to be the supporters in providing livelihood for their parents. In addition to this, in the premodern agrarian setting, mortality, particularly child mortality, was high, hence, the parents had to have a number of children in order to ensure that at least one son would survive to support the life of the parents after their retirement from economic activities. On the other hand, we should consider the cost of raising children to adulthood. In the premodern agrarian societies, the cost of raising children to adulthood is relatively small. In the agrarian societies, education is generally not required, and if it is required, compulsory education is often limited to the grade school level and few children proceed to a higher education. Hence, the balance between the value and cost of children becomes positive and substantial and there are good reasons for having high fertility to ensure the community's and own family's survival.

With the advent of industrialization, urbanization and secularization, the value and cost of children have changed dramatically. In urban and industrial societies, there are no ways in which children can contribute to the economic activities of their parents and households. There are no farms where children can work harvesting crops and there are no blacksmith cottages to which they can bring bales of water and fire logs. Besides, with the arrival of compulsory mass education, children have to go to school in the daytime and, even if parents want to use them for domestic chores and economic activities in the household, children are absent from home and are simply not available to parents. On the other hand, in the context of industrialization, children are required to have higher education through high schools and colleges and universities in order to get decent and high-salaried jobs in offices and factories. The expenses for educating their sons and daughters are rapidly increasing, therefore the balance between the value and cost of having children becomes negative instead of positive and quite substantial. If the net balance between the utility and cost of bearing and rearing children becomes negative (less utility and more cost), then there would be only limited room to have children. If parents still want children, it is because they want the pleasures of home life with their children.

One of the leading demographers of our time, Ansley J. Coale, has suggested three general prerequisites for a major fall in fertility, particularly in marital fertility in the developing countries:[3]

1. Fertility must be considered a matter for rational choice. Couples must both be aware of the possibility of controlling family size and find it an acceptable form of behavior.
2. Reduced fertility must be seen as advantageous within the context of the perceived social and economic circumstances.
3. Effective and acceptable techniques of birth control must be known and accessible.

In many developing countries, condition (1) does not exist. In such countries, children are considered the gift and blessing from God or heaven and the controlling of fertility is blasphemy and sacrilege. The very concept that persons have the right to control their own fertility and can technically do so is not known to many people. At the same time, condition (2) does not apply to most of the people living on agriculture in the developing countries. Again in those agrarian villages, children are producers and at the same time consumers and their services in the household mean important additions to the household labor force to promote production. Secondly, children are the source of the parents' social security in the future. On the other hand, in agrarian settings the cost of raising children is often minimal, hence, the net balance is definitely advantageous for having more children than having less.

And third, on the basis of the above-mentioned conditions, many developing countries promote the import of modern contraceptives, such as the pill and the IUD, from the developed countries, in addition to traditional methods of using condom, diaphragm, jelly, tablets, douche as well as coitus interruptus, etc. As a matter of fact, most countries in South and East Asia and Latin America do not ban free access to those contraceptives among the general public. Mauldin and Lapham have demonstrated that government efforts have played a big role in reducing the crude birth rate in developing countries.[4] The availability of contraceptives and attainment of good population education generally create considerable differences in the actual practice of family planning as has been demonstrated in many cases in the developed countries. We also will discuss this in the next section.

The above-mentioned are the main reasons why fertility in developing countries has been kept high and why the people there usually resist or have not subscribed to the idea of fertility control and family planning in spite of high population growth. In order to get the ball rolling, industrialization and urbanization certainly help to facilitate breaking up the necessity for high fertility in the developing countries. It certainly limits the opportunity of child labor. But government provision of old-age security also would discourage high fertility, along with a general increase in health among the aged. If health is improved among the aged through various preventive medical measures, then most of the aged would not be incapacitated and could work longer at farms and other work places. For example, JOICFP, the Japanese Organization for International Cooperation in Family Planning, reported that in Asia and Africa, practically 100 percent of people in rural areas are infested with parasitic worms, thus having frail vitality in old age. If parasitic worms are eradicated, for example, health is restored, vigor is regained and old people can work more, thus decreasing appreciably the need for social security.

The Situation in the Developed Countries

On the other hand, fertility in the more developed countries is low because the economic activity of children is very low and the cost of raising and giving proper education is very high. As already mentioned, in the urban industrial settings of the developed countries, there is no place at home for children to assist their parents' gainful work in as much as most of the parents work outside home as operatives, office workers and service-rendering workers. Besides, children have to acquire education beyond compulsory education in the developed countries since education is the ticket to enter and get a higher status on the occupational ladder. On the other hand, getting a higher education nowadays has become so costly that parents cannot afford to send more than two children to universities or polytechnical higher schools. Furthermore, the movement towards the liberation of women and provision of equal status for women as much as men has become a sweeping and irreversible trend, seen practically in every country in the developed regions. The labor force participation rates have risen remarkably in those countries not only for unmarried, but also for married women in recent years, and women who have relinquished gainful work in order to bear and rear children have suffered a serious loss of opportunities for career advancement.

In this connection, one has to mention the hostile environment to child-bearing in cities and metropolitan areas in the developed countries. It also should be mentioned that the urban setting, which is characterized by barren monoliths of concrete apartments, by high crime rates and by lack of green spaces and playgrounds for children, is inhibitive to the very existence of children and seems unsuitable for child-bearing activities.

In addition, as already referred to in the previous section, emphasis should be laid upon the widespread availability of highly effective contraceptive technology. The technology of fertility control has improved tremendously in the past 20 years and has been diffused widely throughout the population and among countries. The introduction of oral contraceptives and IUDs around 1962 throughout non-Socialist Europe is considered to have been highly conducive to the precipitous decline in fatalities in Europe in 1964. In the United States, it was reported that the introduction of the pill made a contraceptive revolution by reducing considerably unwanted births among many couples. It is interesting to note that such a contraceptive revolution occurred, even in a country like the United States, where aspirations are high and the means of contraception are thought to have already been widely available.[5] Together with liberalization of induced abortion and availability of safe sterilization, the advent of the contraceptive revolution played an important role in fertility reduction by virtually eliminating unwanted births in the West.

Finally, mention should be made of recent changes in marriage and the family which is also highly related to fertility decline. In recent years, a number of developed countries have been experiencing a revolution in respect of the incidence and timing of legal first marriages. The causes of this revolution are as yet unclear. According to the United Nations 1980 Monitoring Report, however, it seems reasonable to hypothesize that responsible factors include the youth revolution, changes in the status and role of women and, not the least important, the radical changes that have occurred in the efficiency of contraceptives, easier access to them and far wider incidence of their use.

Indeed, in the United States, starting about 1962, the annual rate of divorce rose sharply; it jumped from 9 per 1,000 population in 1960 to 22 per 1,000 in 1979. In Sweden, according to Jan Trost, out of every 100 couples, 15 were unmarried in 1978 and one in three children was born out of wedlock.[6] In the Federal Republic of Germany, between 1965 and 1978, crude birth rate nearly halved from 17.7 to 9.4 per 1,000. Of this decline, about 40 percent is attributable to the marked decline in nuptiality and the remaining 60 percent is accounted for by the phenomenal decrease in marital fertility, particularly among couples with three or more children.

If the above-mentioned aspirations for freedom and enjoyment of an adult-oriented life, the revolution relating to marriage, and a low-fertility syndrome and the other causes for current low fertility in the developed countries are taken into account, it would seem very difficult for governments to introduce pronatalist policies to increase fertility in the developed countries. It might look like a futile effort unless such a philosophical tide and such a life-style change could be thwarted and reversed. It is symbolic, despite the rising concern about the current low-fertility situation. France is the only major country in Northern and Western Europe to have implemented pronatalist population policies with some success.

Consideration of Human Values in Relation to Birth Control

Population growth can be reduced in only three ways: raise mortality, promote migration and lower fertility. The first is, of course, unacceptable and the second unfeasible. Hence, lowered fertility has become an intermediate goal of the development policy in many developing countries. According to the resolutions of past United Nations conferences, all married couples in the world today have the "human right" to have the number of children they want, subject to some appropriate languages about parental responsibility, and moreover, have the legal right as well. However, if a country lacks sufficient land, resources and capital, it is difficult to have any economic take-off, and the sky-high birth rate creates a menace and threat to their capital accumulation at the initial stage for launching industries and for increasing people's overall well-being and welfare. In other words, if the country is caught in a Malthusian trap in which any increase in agricultural production is eaten up by an ever-increasing number of newborn babies, then the government does not have much choice besides taking steps to curb a runaway birth rate and making efforts to disseminate to the people the idea of family planning and the knowledge and methods of practicing family planning.

Although as will be cited later, Julian Simon argues that the ultimate resource is human beings and that any increase in population is a boon to humanity,[7] this idea may be largely applicable only to the United States, Canada and Australia, where there are sufficient land and natural resources, but not pertinent to a country like Bangladesh where the threat of population increase is great and easily offsets the advantages to be gained from population growth. At least as a matter of exigency, fertility control can be justified in Bangladesh, as well as in modern China, the latter of which has been well-known for making efforts to implement a one-child policy. In these countries, national interests may be considered to reasonably override the individual right of freedom and choice. Yet, it should be pointed out that in fact they have been paying serious attention to avoid as much as possible coercion and suppression. It is understood that considerable debate, persuasion and guidance took place, and there was widespread recognition that imminent catastrophe was likely unless action was taken immediately. Imagine that the population growth continues at a rapid rate of nearly two percent and the world population will soon reach 50 billion, 100 billion or to the point where not only amenity in life is lost, but also food shortages, energy crises and pollution are in the offing and would soon decimate the population. The facts that the earth has limits to the availability of its natural resources and limits to its growth are obvious, vis-à-vis population and other forms of economic activity. Are we still capable of talking about human rights and entitlements in this kind of situation? The answer is "yes" though we actually wish to make our answer in a qualified manner.

Coming back to the case of Bangladesh and similar countries

in the developing world, the government should recognize the reasons why some households still tend to have a number of children. They tend to have a number of children because (1) child mortality is high, thus parents should provide a spare person; (2) there is a need for youth labor inasmuch as agriculture requires a lot of labor at the busy seasons of planting and harvesting; and (3) there is no public security system for the aged. If the government needs to introduce national population policies, administrators must consider the above demographic needs, hence, they must make adequate preparation to give security to each household to ensure the well-being of the old, and must teach the need for family planning and the need to reduce the number of children, not by coercion, but through educational explanation of the nation's needs and people's welfare and well-being, as well as reference to quality of life and enhancement of human value. If national interests are to override individual interests, the length of time during which the application of crash program measures is made should be limited to a minimum, and the government should give as much education and as many incentives, as necessary, so that individuals can be motivated to follow the national family planning movement.

The recent Chinese policy has been criticized in many quarters of the world. We all remember the sense of puzzlement we felt when we heard the news that China had launched a one-child policy. We were certainly at first bewildered by their efforts in population engineering and by the abruptness and extremeness of their policy. But no Chinese actually likes the one-child policy and it is obvious that they planned and implement it as a matter of emergency. If the population growth rate as seen 10 years ago had continued, China's population would have increased to much more than one billion, and the nation would have really fallen into the Malthusian trap. Furthermore, great famines would have recurred in China as had occurred last in 1958–1961. The only thing that is regretted now is that the Chinese did not appreciate the problem earlier, before the Marxian industrialism prevailed, emphasizing heavy manufacturing industries in the backyard of each home instead of developments of agriculture and light industries, and instead of taking urgent steps to curtail fertility.

What We Should Do About Valuing Human Life

In 1972, the Club of Rome published its celebrated book entitled *The Limits to Growth* and its doomsday conclusion made a tremendous impact on the intellectual community of the world.[8] The tenets of the book have been criticized strongly by many scholars since they were alleged to ignore the vast ability and promise of science and technology, and were alleged to underestimate the resilient forces of the intellectual power of the human race. It was asked that when the catastrophe was approaching, was it likely that people would just sit around and wait for their downfall without really trying something to alleviate or defer the end of the world? In its review of the book, the Task Force of the World Bank states:

> Can we really believe that most of the population of Detroit could succumb to persistent pollutants without the rest of humanity making any adjustments in its producer-consumer behavior? Humanity faces these problems one-by-one, every year in every era, and keeps making its quiet adjustments. It does not keep accumulating them indefinitely till they make catastrophe inevitable. One does not have to believe in an invisible hand to subscribe to such a society. One has merely to believe in human sanity and its instinct for self-preservation.

In 1981, Julian Simon published his controversial book entitled *The Ultimate Resource.* This book is colored by the author's unique optimism in contrast to the pessimism expressed in *The Limits to Growth.* According to Simon, there are virtually no limits to natural resources, even to energy resources which have been considered most exhaustible. When there are advancements in science and technology, humankind will not face the resource scarcity and population problems. Population increase promotes economic growth. Necessity is the mother for innovation and new devices. He concludes that for most of the relevant economic matters he has checked, the trends are positive rather than negative. And he doubts that it does the troubled people of the world any good to say that things are getting worse though they are really getting better. The major fuel to speed our progress is our stock of knowledge, and the brake is our lack of imagination. The ultimate resource is people—skilled, spirited and hopeful people who will exert their wills and imaginations for their benefits, and so, inevitably, for the benefit of us all.

The philosophy of Julian Simon seems bright, rosy and very promising. It seems to us, however, that it depends on the type of country in which you live. If you live in a country like the United States, Canada or Australia, where resources and land are plentiful, then you can certainly exert your will and imagination to generate better living conditions and a greater population may promote economic development. It is true in human history that population expansion generally pushes further economic development. But what about Bangladesh, the Philippines, India, Korea, Costa Rica, Panama and even China today? The mere man-land ratio and the lack of natural resources, together with the lack of capital and traditional society, stifle any imagination. Imagination alone cannot promote economic development and prosperity. Extreme poverty, filth and overcrowding, due to the lack of natural resource, heavy population density and the fatalistic way of looking at the world reflecting such geodemographic situations, simply suffocates the people's will to strive for a better life. The value of human life, though it is very important in an abstract sense, often becomes meaningless and worthless under extremely severe and poor circumstances. Human dignity and human value can only be restored by economic development through curbing population growth.

It is true that the Club of Rome report on *The Limits to Growth* is certainly overpessimistic and underestimates the role to be played by science and technology and human volition. One can ask that since science and technology cannot control street crimes, traffic jams and accidents, housing shortages, or stagflation, how can it cope with the increasing population and deteriorating environmental conditions in the world—desertification, soil erosion, acid rain, increase of carbon monoxide in the air, etc.? Nevertheless, we still believe that science and technology can at least postpone considerably the arrival of catastrophe, in some cases for several hundred years instead of two or three decades implied in *The Limits to Growth.*

But then, after all, the resources contained in the earth are not unlimited and in the ultimate future they will be depleted and exhausted. The earth is the limit. To repeat, science and technology can only postpone the arrival of the end of the world, but cannot eliminate the prospect of catastrophe. If the present rate of consumption continues to grow along with the population growth, it must finally face resource depletion and exhaustion even though fertility is rapidly declining. Human society might survive for 500 years, but probably not beyond that. To the Spaceship called Earth, rapid population growth cannot continue on forever, but must cease at some point and some time. Although each additionally born child may be a blessing from the god to the parents, it is not necessarily the case that a newborn baby is always welcome to its surrounding world or represents a strong case of human value.

Concluding Remarks

It is very difficult to think about the value of human life in many developing countries. Extreme poverty, filth and downgraded human conditions in these countries represent a kind of human pollution and shame to human kind. It is difficult to conceive human dignity in an extremely crowded and poverty-stricken situation. In the morning rush hour in Japan, where people are packed in suburban trains or subway cars just like sardines, there are only masses of human flesh and bones, not human spirit. There can be no human dignity for people who do not even have a standing space under foot in the train. And, in a country like Bangladesh, an enormous population increase simply aggravates the living conditions of the people and gives no prospect of improving their standard of living. Worst of all, the people have accepted and acquiesced such a kind of situation by asking what else they can do.

The present writer believes that there is a real emergency or crisis and that some fundamental measures should be taken immediately. The family planning movement is, perhaps, the way to emancipate humankind from hunger, misery, indignity and lack of respect, and to restore the value of human life.

The fundamental measures thus mentioned include two avenues: the first being a crash-program for the governments to support and spread rapidly to the general public, in birth control and family planning. If people have no idea or knowledge of family planning, then the idea and philosophy of why women should practice it has to be emphasized. Teaching and persuasion, instead of coercion, should be employed. Prior to persuasion and guidance, population education in school is important to lay down the foundation for efficient implementation and practice of family planning programs. The second avenue includes economic development, increase in the standard of living, enhancement of education and elimination of illiteracy. Certainly, development is often considered better than contraceptives. But its drawback is slowness; often you cannot wait another 50 years to attain a low birth rate or a low growth rate of population. Some quick emergency measures are required. Nobody wants to take bitter pills, but under the present circumstances of many developing countries, fundamental and farsighted measures are needed to recover and establish firmly the value of human life.

NOTES

1. Thomas Robert Malthus, *An Essay on the Principle of Population* (London: Johnson, 1798).

2. Norman E. Himes, *Medical History of Contraception* (New York: Gamut Press, Inc., 1963).

3. A.J. Coale, "The Demographic Transition," International Union for the Scientific Study of Population, *International Population Conference*, Leige, 1973, vol.1, 53–73.

4. W. Parker Mauldin and Bernard Berelson, "Conditions of Fertility Decline in Developing Countries, 1965–75," *Studies in Family Planning*, vol. 9, no. 5, 1978.

5. Charles F. Westoff and Norman Ryder, *The Contraceptive Revolution* (Princeton: Princeton University Press, 1977).

6. Jan Trost, "Dissolution of Cohabitation and Marriage in Sweden," *Journal Of Divorce*, vol. 2, Summer 1979, 415–421.

7. Julian L. Simon, *The Ultimate Resource* (Princeton: Princeton University Press, 1981).

8. Donella H. Meadows, Dennis L. Meadows, Jorgen Randers and William W. Behrens III, *The Limits to Growth* (New York: Universe Books, 1972).

9. Julian Simon, *The Ultimate Resource.*

SIX

HOW PEOPLE ARGUE ABOUT ABORTION And CAPITAL PUNISHMENT

IN EUROPE AND AMERICA AND WHY

Christie Davies

During the second half of the 20th century, two phenomena involving the evaluation of human life *viz.* abortion and capital punishment have been the subject of much controversy. These controversies have tended to be settled in a particular direction. In most of the countries of the Western world[1] (and many others as well), capital punishment has been abolished or its use radically reduced and restricted and the law relating to abortion considerably liberalized, thus permitting a significant rise in the number of legal (as distinct from clandestine) abortions.

Among the more recent Western countries to abolish capital punishment have been Australia (Commonwealth) (1968), Austria (1968), Canada (1974), France (1981), Spain (1979), Switzerland (1974), and the United Kingdom (1965).[2] The United States is now the only major Western democracy to retain capital punishment, but even so there has been a marked decline in its use, despite a rising incidence of violent "capital" crimes, and between 1967 and 1977 no executions took place.

TABLE 6-1[3]	
Years	Number of persons executed under civil authority in the United States
1935–1939	891
1940–1944	645
1950–1954	413
1955–1959	304
1960–1964	181
1965–1969	10
1970–1980	3

The common trend in relation to abortion is even more striking and, indeed, more extensive. By 1979, two-thirds of the world's population lived in countries where abortion was legal and obtainable either on request or for a broad range of social as well as medical reasons (and in yet others, laws prohibiting abortion are no longer enforced). In 1971, less than 40 percent of the world's population were living in countries with this degree of deregulation.[4] In particular, the main Western industrial countries have nearly all adopted relatively liberal abortion laws, as can be seen from Table 6-2.

It also should be noted that all the other Scandinavian countries now have enacted extremely liberal abortion laws and that abortion is de facto freely available in the Netherlands and Scotland.[6] Also, women who are resident in the few European countries with more restrictive legislation on abortion freely (and in large numbers) obtain abortions in adjoining countries. Thus, Ireland's abortions are performed in Britain and Belgian women

TABLE 6-2[5]

Country	Dates of major liberalizations of the abortion laws
Austria	1974
Denmark	1970; 1973
England and Wales	1967
France	1975
Germany (West)	1974; 1976
Italy	1978
Luxembourg	1978
U.S.A.	1973 (earlier in some states)

obtain abortions in the Netherlands.[7] In 1979, Mme. Monique Pelletier, the French Minister for Family Affairs, speaking at a European conference on abortion laws held in Paris, noted that attitudes to abortion and the law were converging throughout Western Europe[8] (with the exception of Ireland) and this has continued to be the case.

It is the author's aim to examine this convergence of the laws relating to capital punishment and to abortion in the Western democracies and to suggest reasons for these parallel changes. The main evidence will be taken from a detailed examination of the arguments employed in the British Parliament at the time that the relevant legal reforms took place. In general, the changes that occurred in Britain and the arguments used to legitimize them may be taken as typical of the other West European countries and indeed of many of the individual states of the United States of America and can be linked to other broad social changes occurring throughout the Western industrial countries. However, in the United States, as a whole, the execution of liberal abortion and the aborting of liberal execution took place by a different route and were legitimized by appeals to a different set of values. Americans involved in these changes came to argue about abortion and capital punishment in ways radically different from their British and West European counterparts, in part because of the nature of the American Constitution and in part because of the distinctively moralistic quality of American culture.

From Moralism to Causalism

During the decade 1959–1969, the British Parliament passed a number of important Private Members Bills [bills promoted by individual Members of Parliament (M.P's), as distinct from the government, and on which the members enjoy a "free" vote undirected by the leaders of their particular Party], dealing with such controversial moral issues as illegitimacy (1959), Obscene Publications (1959), Capital Punishment(1965), (Homo)Sexual Offenses (1967), Abortion (1967), Theater Censorship (1968) and Divorce (1969).[9] The law in each of these areas traditionally embraced a particular moral outlook which I have termed "moralism," and this was also the moral creed of those who opposed reform of these laws. By contrast, the successful law reformers adhered to a very different set of moral principles and assumptions that I have termed "causalism." For the moralist, it is a good and sufficient reason to forbid an activity (such as abortion, homosexual behavior, the publication of pornography) and to punish those detected in it if their actions can be represented as wrong in themselves, as immoral or wicked, quite regardless of the consequences of the acts themselves or of attempts to forbid them by law. The purpose of the law is to identify the guilty and the innocent, to penalize the former and protect the latter, to reward the virtuous and to punish the wicked with suitable severity up to, and including, the taking of a guilty life for a sufficiently heinous offense such as murder, rape, treason or collaboration with an enemy army of occupation. It is not, however, a merely restrictive moral outlook, for it can incorporate or at least take cognizance of libertarian assertions of a person's right to be free to order his or her own life (provided he or she does not transgress the basic moral rules laid down by the moralists), even if the consequences of such behavior are harmful to the actor or a nuisance to others. By contrast, "causalists" are not primarily concerned with individual virtues and vices or even motives but with questions of cause and consequence. If it turns out that more harm is done by using the law to forbid an activity than by allowing it, then causalists will be willing to permit it, even if they consider such behavior to be immoral or wicked. Whereas the aim of the moralist is to distribute benefits and penalties according to the moral deserts of the parties involved in a situation, causalists seek merely to minimize the overall harm and suffering experienced by the various people concerned, regardless of their moral status or past behavior. The moralist pursues justice; the causalist seeks welfare. Causalists are essentially short-term negative utilitarians. They will choose to exact or repeal a law, not to maximize happiness or the excess of happiness over suffering but to minimize suffering which for them is the greatest of human evils. They are in no sense hedonists or visionaries—they are only concerned with present disutility, with the avoidance of today's tangible but visible suffering, distress, harm and conflict.

The above definitions and descriptions are ideal types, abstracted and constructed from the arguments employed in British parliamentary debates and reports on nonparty issues, such as capital punishment and abortion. It is to these debates we must now turn for an examination of the profound changes that have occurred in the way British legislators argue about moral issues.

Arguing About Abortion in Britain

The supporters of the Medical Termination of Pregnancy Bill of 1966, which in an amended form became the Abortion Act of 1967, put forward a predominantly causalist case stressing the stark alternative sets of consequences. They did not put forward a case for liberty or privacy, nor for women's rights to command their own bodies and to be free from state-enforced control over their sexuality. They simply insisted that legalized abortion was the lesser of two evils.[10]

The reformers' case was repeatedly presented in terms of the need to clarify and extend the law relating to abortion so that the dangerous practices of illicit and often unqualified, medically ignorant abortionists could be replaced by the careful technique of qualified doctors licensed by the state, even if this meant openly permitting and implicitly condoning an activity previously regarded as morally abhorrent. The reformers repeatedly stressed the immediate and specific issues involved and the limited number of likely alternative outcomes available to or possible for unwillingly pregnant women. The wider moral, philosophical and religious issues were played and controversial assertions of rights and values avoided. Cause and consequence was all.

The reformers' tactics created a dilemma for those who opposed any liberalization of the then existing law which permitted abortion if continued pregnancy would place the mother's life at risk, or (on the basis of a case law precedent the Bourne judgment) seriously endanger her health. They clearly found abortion morally repugnant, yet they realized that they could not successfully oppose reform of the law on this basis in a predominantly causalist legislature.[11]

The causalist nature of Britain's reform of the abortion laws is best illustrated by contrasting the essentially causalist final wording of the Abortion Act that became law, with the moralists clauses and amendments relating to rape victims and to underage or mentally defective mothers which were rejected by Parliament. In essence, the law of 1967 declared that abortion was permissible when in the view of the relevant doctors, (a) "the continuance of the pregnancy would involve risk to the life of the pregnant woman, or of injury to the physical and mental health of the pregnant woman or any existing children or her family greater than if the pregnancy were terminated." In making this determination, the doctors may take account of "the pregnant woman's actual or reasonably foreseeable environment." Or (b) "there is a substantial risk that if the child were born it would suffer from such physical and mental abnormalities as to be seriously handicapped."[12]

The British Abortion Act of 1967 makes no reference to rights or just desert. Abortion is permitted if it will prevent mental and physical suffering on the part of the woman concerned and, indeed, her existing children whether the causes of this be medical, social or psychological.

Some of those moralists in Parliament who were strongly opposed to abortion nonetheless tried unsuccessfully to amend the Abortion Bill to permit abortion in the case of rape, i.e., they believed that abortion should be granted on the basis of the moral deserts of the mother rather than her propensity for suffering. On this view the fetus ought not to be destroyed because it is *innocent* (a key word in the moralists' lexicon), but its special moral status may be disregarded and its rights may be set aside if the mother can assert an equal claim to innocence as in the case of the pregnant victim of a rapist. The Conservative Member of

Parliament, Mrs. Jill Knight, found abortion abhorrent, but was prepared to allow this abhorrence to be overridden by her even greater abhorrence of rape.

The thrust of Mrs. Knight's argument is that the woman who has been raped deserves an abortion, not because she is liable to suffer a great deal of harm, but because she is free of all blame.[13] The sexual act which had led to conception was unwilled, involuntary, forced upon her and thus she falls in the most deserving of the moralists' categories—she is a victim.

Indeed, Simms and Hindel describe the opponents of a further liberalization of the law relating to abortion as often being strongly convinced that abortion should be reserved for the virtuous:

> The Rev. K. Ward, Rector of Daventry…told (his congregation) that as Christians they must be certain that abortion was not "made available for all and sundry who behave promiscuously and irresponsibly." This notion that abortion, if it was to be tolerated at all, should be a reward for virtue, whereas the wicked and irresponsible should be punished with unwanted babies was a recurrent theme throughout the SPUC (Society for the Protection of the Unborn Child) campaign and was probably the attitude most often voiced in the campaign against reform.[14]

It was, however, an attitude that badly divided the opponents of abortion, for the view that abortions should be granted to the virtuous and innocent was anathema to other moralists who felt it was even more unjust to penalize the innocent fetus for the misdeeds of the guilty rapist.[15]

These divisions within the moralist camp were largely irrelevant since the reformers had taken control of the culturally dominant causalist view of abortion. David Steel's original Bill contained a clause permitting abortion after rape, but he shrewdly withdrew it as a result of causalist criticisms and opposed attempts to reintroduce such a clause:

> I hope that the Hon. Member will not press the Amendment because I believe that the cases of genuine sexual assault and unlawful carnal knowledge are catered for by the discretion given to the medical profession to consider these two matters regarding the total environment of the patient and her mental health.[16]

The British Parliament rejected the rape clause and also amendments that would have granted an abortion automatically where the pregnant woman was under 16 or mentally defective. As in the case of rape, these pregnancies also would have been the result of a criminal offense since the woman could not in any real sense be said to have given her consent. The pregnant young girl or mental defective can be regarded as "innocents," as victims of circumstances outside their control or capacity for control. However, the lawmakers insisted that the key criterion was one of harm to the mother or her family and not guilt or innocence. It was argued that the problems of the "innocents," of the cretinous (crétin is derived from Chrétien and refers to the innocence of idiocy), did not deserve separate and special consideration because of their distinctive moral status.

The shift from restrictive abortion laws perceived as (i.e., regardless of the particular balance of factors that had led to their original enactment)[17] based on a moralist principle to more liberal laws justified on causalist grounds can be seen most clearly in the case of the changes that took place in England and Wales, but the model also is applicable to the process of reform that has taken place in other West European countries and also (during the period 1965–1973)[18] in several individual American states. Thus, the realization that the laws prohibiting abortion were unenforceable and led to a high incidence of suffering by women who died or became ill as a result of botched clandestine abortions at the hands of unskilled abortionists considerably influenced opinion in France and Italy. In France, the right-wing president, Giscard d'Estaing,[19] argued strongly for a new law that took account of this harsh reality, and the political parties supporting the liberalization of the abortion laws in Italy strongly stressed the need to replace back-street abortions with safe legal procedures at the time of the Italian referenda on the subject.[20] This argument also was pressed strongly by those campaigning for legislative change in individual American states. [21]

The contents of the more liberal laws introduced in Europe[22] and in those American states that changed their laws prior to the Supreme Court decision of 1973 are reasonably similar to that of the legislation of England and Wales. It should be noted, though, that whereas, of the major European countries, only in Germany does the law specifically mention rape or felonious intercourse as a ground for granting an abortion (French and Italian law do not), most of those American states that reformed their laws specified forcible rape, statutory rape and incest as reasons for permitting consequent abortion.[23] In many cases this may have been because the legislators adopted all or part of the section of the American Law Institute's Model Penal Code,[24] dealing with abortion. Whether or not this was the case, the difference between America and Europe in this respect is a mark of the much more strongly "moralist" culture of America.

From Moralism to Causalism: The Case of Capital Punishment

The debates that have taken place in the British Parliament on the subject of capital punishment have thrown up moralist and causalist arguments on both sides. Among those who were in favor of retaining the death penalty were moralists, who saw it as a just retribution for the crime of murder or as a means of witnessing to society's moral abhorrence of such an evil crime through the solemn emphatic ritual denunciation and condemnation of the murderer by means of the sentence of execution and the execution of that sentence. Others were causalists who believed, or said they believed, that the fear of the death penalty deters those who are tempted to murder another. Among the abolitionists were those who saw the death penalty, the deliberate judicial taking of human life by the state, as so wrong in principle that it should never be used, regardless of whether or not it deters murderers (or in other jurisdictions, rapists, muggers or drug traffickers.) Other abolitionists saw the very existence of the death penalty as having a harmful effect on society in general, as having a morbid or inflammatory effect on the attitudes and imaginings of the ordinary citizen. There were also causalists among the ranks of the abolitionists—those who regard the death penalty as an ineffective deterrent (i.e., no more effective than other less drastic penalties) or even as an incentive to commit murder for a few bizarre and possibly suicidal exhibitionists, or for those who calculate that the existence of the death penalty makes juries less willing to convict. An issue also raised by the abolitionists, which has both a moralist and causalist dimension, was the possibility that an error in the course of a trial[25] for a capital crime could lead to a guiltless person being executed. The moralist abolitionist is troubled by the thought that an *innocent* person might be *unjustly* penalized beyond all possibility of compensation. Causalists, in general, tend to dislike *irreversible* measures which are incompatible with their ethic of responsibility rather than absolute ends and which leave no room for a change of mind in the light of new evidence regarding relative consequences.

The history of the balance of these different arguments in relation to capital punishment is a complex one, but it may very roughly be said that over time Britain's abolitionists changed from being moralist humanitarian crusaders to be causalist reformers emphasizing cause and consequence.[26] Similarly, there was a decline in the popularity or acceptability of retribution as a theme and those who supported capital punishment in Parliament came to argue for it very largely on the basis of its deterrent value.

The change can perhaps best be illustrated by looking at the period since World War II. In 1948, the members of the House of Commons on a free vote added a clause suspending the death penalty for five years to the Labor Government's Criminal Justice Bill. The House of Lords, acting in the view of the peers as the will of the people,[27] deleted the clause, and the government, in order to rescue its original bill, instructed Labor M.P.'s to vote for it as amended by the Lords. The debates were characterized by a more full-blooded assertion of moralist views on both sides than was customary in the decades that followed.[28]

These strongly moralist views for and against capital punishment flourished at this time in part at least because of the fervor and intensified group loyalties stimulated by the events of World War II and its aftermath. Indeed, this fact was recognized by many of those who took part in the debates.[29]

The effect of the war on the use of capital punishment in Europe was even greater than the British Parliamentarians had thought. In the defeated nations of Italy and Germany (Federal Republic), capital punishment was abolished because it symbolized that power of the state to execute which had been so misused under the Fascist and National Socialist regimes. In Italy, the death penalty for civil offenses was abolished in 1944 by legislative decree after the downfall of Mussolini.[30] In the Federal Republic of Germany, the death penalty was abolished in 1949 as part of the basic law of the new Federal Republic that succeeded the Third Reich.[31] (The state's right to execute does, however, live on in East Germany.)

A moralist movement in the opposite direction occurred in Denmark, Luxembourg and the Netherlands, where the death penalty was reintroduced in order to execute collaborators and war criminals.[32] A sleeping death penalty was reactivated for essentially similar reasons in Belgium, Norway and Israel.[33] In all these cases, capital punishment was brought back as an act of retributive justice, as a statement of society's collective identity and values and of the rightful power of the state to assert the overriding importance of these things by taking the lives of those men and women who had transgressed against them.

In Britain, as Leslie Hale predicted, idealism gave way to empiricism. The report of the Royal Commission on Capital Punishment 1949–1953 is a sober document much concerned with assessing the strength or weakness of the argument that capital punishment is a unique deterrent by analyzing relevant data from other European and Commonwealth countries and from the individual states of the United States.[34] At the core of its deliberations lie considerations of cause (hence, my neologism "causalism") and consequence. Retribution, reprobation, atonement and expiation occupy a very minor place in the report and, indeed, there are explicit comments on the declining regard for such factors in penological thought.[35]

A full triumph of the causalist ethic can be seen in the Conservative Government's Homicide Act of 1957, which abolished capital punishment for certain categories of murder but retained it for others. The division between capital and noncapital murder in this British Act of 1957 is much more clearly and emphatically causalist than is the case with the distinctions between first and second-degree murder to be found historically in many American states and, indeed, in earlier unsuccessful legislative proposals in Britain itself.[36] It is certainly far more consistently causalist than the sections of the American Law Institute's *Moral Penal Code* relating to capital punishment of approximately the same date (Draft No. 9, 1959).[37]

The 1957 Act imposed the death penalty for certain categories of murder only, not because they were "especially heinous, atrocious or cruel, manifesting exceptional depravity,"[38] but because it was postulated that murderers of this kind were the most likely to be deterred from killing by the threat of execution. The capital murders were: killing in the course of theft, the killing of policemen and prison officers, killing by shooting (most people in Britain do not own or keep guns in their homes) or an explosion, and the committing of murders on separate occasions.[39] These were seen as instrumental, "rational" murders as a means to an end by criminals who were presumed to calculate the rewards and penalties involved in any criminal enterprise that might involve killing. This was in contrast to the impulsive murders of other family members or close associates in the course of a quarrel or as a result of an unbearable emotional situation. Certain types of murders generally thought to be especially vile and culpable now no longer carried the death penalty—sex murders, the murder of innocent children, poisoning and parricide were all non-capital offenses.

In 1965, the British retentionists finally lost the argument about deterrence. In particular, there had been very little difference between the trends of capital and of non-capital murder in the years following the introduction of this distinction in 1957. The abolitionists were able to cast sufficient doubt on the retentionists' central assumption that capital punishment was a unique deterrent to enable them to win a majority for abolition in *both* Houses of Parliament.

The abolitionists, knowing that they were not winning the causalist arguments, are apparently willing to concede the moral reasonableness of the deterrence argument criticizing it only in terms of its factual inaccuracy. Henry Brooke's conversion to abolitionism was particularly interesting since as Home Secretary in an earlier Conservative Government he had upheld capital punishment but had now changed his mind regarding the facts of deterrence.[40]

The situation since 1965 has remained unchanged. In 1970 (i.e. five years after 1965) a Parliament with a Labor majority confirmed and made permanent the provisional five-year abolition of capital punishment of 1965. In 1983, in a Parliament with a large Conservative majority, attempts to restore capital punishment for all murders, or more narrowly for the murder of police officers, of prison officers, for murder by shooting or causing an explosion, for murder in the furtherance of theft and for terrorist murders all failed by a substantial margin of votes.[41]

The evolution of views of capital punishment in the British Parliament may then be summed up roughly as in Figures 6-1 and 6-2 below.

FIGURE 6-1

	Moralists ──────────→ Causalists	
Retentionists and Restorers	Capital punishment is just retribution for and salutary denunciation of the willful and unlawful taking of human life ──→	Capital punishment deters murderers and on balance reduces suffering and loss of life
Abolitionists	Capital punishment is always wrong. It has a harmful effect on society and devalues human life.	Capital punishment is an ineffective deterrent and thus involves an unjustifiable taking of life and infliction of suffering.

FIGURE 6-2

	Moralists ──────────→ Causalists	
Retained	Traditional mandatory capital punishment for murder ──────→	Homicide Act of 1957 Capital punishment for "deterable" murders
Abolished	Thwarted attempt at abolition 1948	Abolition - 1965 Confirmed - 1970 Failure of attempt at restoration - 1983

Moralism, Causalism, Abortion and Capital Punishment in Britain

I have argued above that a fundamental shift has occurred in the way key issues about the value of human are discussed in Britain by those who have the power to implement their views. In part this is because sincere moralists have given way to sincere causalists (either through replacement or conversion) and in part because moralists in Parliament who wish to persuade others or to retain credibility are forced to make use of causalists' arguments and reasoning. The question of which M.P.'s is, however, a matter of interest only to social psychologists. For the sociologist it is enough to note that the *dominant* form of moral argument changed over time. Causalism became dominant as more members of Parliament came to view moral issues in this way and as it became dominant, other members felt obliged to make their public arguments conform to the causalist framework. For some, causalism is a definite pattern of moral belief, for others a tactic they must adopt, possibly at times in bad faith. It is doubtful though whether much would be gained by adopting an alternative analysis that would regard public argument as a mere epiphenomenal superstructure to be cast aside in a hunt for Paretian residues, unconscious motives, hidden agendas or underlying material interests. Indeed, some of the most interesting insights into the conflicting evaluations of the importance of human life expressed in the Parliamentary debates stem from the inability of sincere moralists and sincere causalists to understand one another's point of view. This is particularly evident in the clashes and misunderstandings that occurred between moralists who were in favor of capital punishment and of restrictive abortion laws and causalists who wanted to abolish capital punishment and liberalize the law relating to abortion. The Conservative M.P. Mrs. Jill Knight, a strongly moralist member of the former camp, genuinely found the latter point of view quite perplexing:

> Once we accept that it is lawful to kill a human being because it causes inconvenience, where do we end? Society, or at any rate the majority in this House, has already conceded that the life of a convicted murderer shall be preserved. How can we possibly agree to that and yet kill the most innocent of things, an unborn baby? It just does not seem to be logical.[42]

There is, of course, a logical consistency in the position of those causalists who both supported the abortion act and sought the abolition of capital punishment, but their moral premises are so different from those of their moralist opponents that communication and comprehension are endangered. In all situations, the causalists wish to avoid harm and reduce suffering, regardless of

114

the moral standing of the participants. For such causalists, the fetus can be sacrificed but not the murderer because its capacity for suffering is less. The fetus cannot anticipate the moment of its demise and cannot experience the mental torture which the condemned man is liable to suffer, a torment that magnifies, concentrates and symbolizes the existential torment of life itself.

Unlike the murderer, the fetus has no plans, expectations, relationships to be suddenly, finally and irreversibly disrupted. It cannot know the sufferings that spring from human self-consciousness and awareness. Also, when a fetus is aborted no one else need to be hurt, whereas an execution can fill those who are attached to the condemned person with a lasting sense of grief and shame. To have a loved sibling executed must be a searing experience. To have an unformed sibling preserved in a pickle-bottle for medical students to gawk at is neither here nor there.

For the moralists, this line of causalist argument was incomprehensible. For them, the elimination of suffering was not the central, indeed overwhelming, goal it was for the causalists but rather something that must be endured in the service of morality and inflicted in the pursuit of justice. The murderer is guilty of taking life, so his or her own life is forfeited; the fetus is innocent, the very symbol of innocence as a preborn babe, and thus sacred.

The American Experience

Much of what I have written above about Britain (and other Western countries) was and is also true of the United States. The liberalization of the abortion laws in individual states prior to the 1973 Supreme Court decision tended to be justified on causalist grounds and the debates about capital punishment became increasingly causalist-utilitarian in character.[43] Deterrence displaced the use of Biblical retributionism as the central retentionist argument and the use of sophisticated methods to test the efficacy of capital punishment as a deterrent (plus the fierce controversies this has aroused) are an index of the central importance of this causalist theme in America.[44] Nonetheless, moralist modes of argument are a more essential part of American than of British discourse and perhaps always have been, ever since the Pilgrim Fathers left England in order to implement the conflicting values of freedom and enforced righteousness in the New World. The

American Constitution is a moralist document and has become a sacred, though secular text used to resolve 20th century dilemmas of law and morality that neither the founding fathers nor later amenders of the Constitution could have envisaged. Though there is a clear separation of church and state in the U.S.A., there is also a greater intensity of popular religious and moral zeal[45] than in any other Western country, except the two Irelands, and there has been a corresponding willingness to make the criminal law the witness and guardian of the community's zealousness. Prohibition, the early antics of the Federal Bureau of Narcotics, Comstock and the Blue Laws, modern anti-porn crusades, the savage punishment of unnatural vice, and the persecution of the early Mormon polygamists are but a few of the historical reminders of American willingness to try to enforce morality by law, thus creating victimless crimes. Many of America's most intense moral conflicts have involved the clash of two distinctively American moralist traditions: (a) the secular assertion of rights and liberties in the Constitution and (b) waves of popular moral fervor rooted in religion that have impelled state and sometimes federal legislators to try to control private individual conduct by law.

Attempts to abolish or to restrict capital punishment or to liberalize or repeal restrictive abortion laws in America at first proceeded on a state-by-state basis, employing essentially causalist arguments within individual State legislatures.[46] However, this proved a slow and uncertain process and ran into increasing opposition from aroused moralists.[47] Individual state legislators, concerned about reselection and reelection, preferred to do nothing rather than risk the wrath of a vocal and aroused moralist opposition among the electorate. British M.P.s by contrast, operate within a much more centralized political system with more strongly organized political parties and a less insistent tradition of populist democracy. In Britain, Nigel Nicholson's Conservative constituency party strongly attacked him because of his support for the abolition of capital punishment,[48] and homosexual reform cost Humphrey Berkeley (Conservative) his seat after an unofficial whispering campaign against him. But these were rare cases. In general, Labor M.P.'s need only fear infiltration of their local party by the extreme left, and Conservative M.P.'s the revelation of personal scandal as possible causes of deselection.

M.P.'s know that at a general election the electors will vote for a particular political party and not for or against the stance of an individual candidate on moral issues. John Parker, the Labor M.P. for Dagenham and a well-known freethinker, prominent in the "liberal" reforms of the 1960s, told the author that attempts to mobilize Roman Catholic votes against him because of his activities had no impact at all on his enormous majority. The blue-collar Roman Catholics working for Ford had their hearts on the right but their wallets were on the left. In the United States, senators can sometimes enjoy a similar degree of independence on moral issues, but congressmen do not and members of the state legislatures which have constitutional responsibility for much "moral" legislation are possibly the most vulnerable of all to the hostility of single groups. Their support won't help a candidate win, but their enmity could ensure that he or she loses, and this often leads legislators to indulge in ambiguous procrastination which favors the status quo and a tyranny not of the majority but of the moral majority.

Faced with a stalemate in the state legislature, the reformers brought a series of cases to the attention of the Supreme Court and it was this body that made the key decisions regarding capital punishment and abortion in America. However, the arguments that were put before the Supreme Court had to be tailored: (a) to the fact that the Court is a judicial body adjudicating on questions of constitutional law and not a legislature; (b) to the particular values and principles enshrined in the American Constitution. Such arguments are of necessity largely moralist in form and the fact that particular moralist arguments were presented before a body that when so persuaded had the power to implement radical social change to freeze the present into immobility or to reverse a historical trend, gave the said moralist arguments a high standing in the general moral discourse of the entire society.

We can thus pinpoint the institutional forces that determine the choice of argument on a particular issue. However, this is inevitable and not necessarily reprehensible. In all societies (or multinational institutions), certain bodies are vested with the authority (i.e., the legitimate power) to make decisions about law and thus about the forceful implementation of measures that are the subject of ethical controversy. In Britain, the doctrine of Parliamentary sovereignty, in America the Constitution determines who the final arbiter shall be and this has a strong influence on the choice of arguments used by pressure groups and activists, who after all are not concerned with scoring philosophic points but with the art of the possible. Any democratic institution that has been vested with the authority to make practical decisions involving the use of the power of the state is constrained in the kinds of argument it can accept or use, either by a written constitution or (as in Britain) by long established constitutional conventions. Also, there are other less choate sets of assumptions operating (a kind of institutional *zeitgeist*) which influence Supreme Court justices or members of Parliament to accept and employ the same forms of argument in relation to morally contentious issues that they make use of when other more mundane questions are being decided.

The American Supreme Court, Abortion and Capital Punishment

In the United States, the key decisions of the Supreme Court that altered the laws of all the states in relation to abortion were made in adjudicating the cases of *Roe v. Wade* (1973) and *Doe v. Bolton* (1973) [later qualified by *Beal v. Doe* (1977), *Maher v. Roe* (1977) and *Harris v. McRae* (1980)]. In the case of capital punishment, the crucial cases were *Furman v. Georgia* (1972), *Woodson v. North Carolina* (1976), *Gregg v. Georgia* (1976), *Harry Roberts v. Louisiana* (1977) and *Coker v. Georgia* (1977). It is to the arguments employed in these judgments that we must now turn.

In the two abortion cases of 1973, the Supreme Court ruled that a state could not intervene in the abortion decision between a woman and her doctor in the first three months of pregnancy and only in order to enact regulations to protect maternal health during the second trimester. Only during the last three months, when the fetus may be assumed to be more or less viable, may a state now prohibit abortion in order to promote potential human life and even then not where an abortion is necessary to preserve the mother's life or health.[49] The Court's decisions swept away all the states' existing laws restricting abortion. The main ground was a moralist assertion of the woman's *right* to privacy:

> This right of privacy, whether it be founded in the Fourteenth Amendment's concept of personal liberty and restrictions upon state action as we feel it is, or as the District Court determined in the Ninth Amendment's reservation of rights to the people, is broad enough to encompass a woman's decision whether or not to terminate her pregnancy.[50]

The key test is the due process clause of the Fourteenth Amendment of the U.S. Constitution:

> nor shall any state deprive any person of life, liberty or property, without due process of law.

Neither here nor elsewhere is a right to privacy as such specifically spelled out, but earlier decisions of the Court on other issues had declared such a right to be implicit in the Constitution and the relevant amendments. The central concern of the Constitution always has been to create boundaries to the power that government has to restrict the liberties of the individual and a right to privacy is a corollary of this concern for liberty and for the "moral primacy of the private over the public sphere of society."[51]

The Supreme Court's decision then was a strongly moralist assertion of women's right to liberty and privacy, even though it was made clear that the woman's right over her own body was not an absolute right but a limited right to be balanced against competing interests. The causalist argument that was at the heart of the British and European debate about abortion was dealt with only indirectly when the Court noted that: "The detriment that the state would impose upon the pregnant woman by denying this choice altogether is apparent"[52] and outlined the medical, psychological, economic and social harms that she was thereby liable to suffer. However, there was little discussion of medical or social science data[53] and the Court clearly saw its area of expertise as limited to legal and constitutional issues, questions of fact or cause and effect being a matter for legislators to resolve.

The American Supreme Court, like the British Parliament, avoided any lengthy discussion of fundamental philosophical and religious doctrines relating to abortion. Parliament had avoided the question of the status and rights (if any) of the fetus by discussing abortion within a framework of pragmatic causalism. The Supreme Court did so by considering the status of the fetus only within the limited perspective of the historical development of Anglo-American common law and of American statute and constitutional law. The moralist claims of those who sought to retain restrictions on abortion in order to uphold the rights of the fetus were rejected by the Court on the grounds that (a) for much of American (and before that English) history, abortion had been tolerated, i.e., the fetus had not been regarded as a "person" entitled to the protection of the laws and the Constitution and (b) the fetus was not regarded as a person for other legal purposes.[54]

The legal arguments in the Supreme Court regarding the death penalty also have tended to be centered on *moralist* questions relating to individual rights viz. "Is the death penalty an inherently cruel and unusual form of punishment?" Can the laws prescribing capital punishment be framed and administered in such a way as not to deprive defendants of their constitutional guarantees of "due process of law" (i.e., trials and appeals characterized by fairness and rule-bound procedural justice) and "equal protection of the laws" (i.e., equal and uniform treatment of all like-situated individuals). The central values appealed to by the opponents of capital punishment were those of fairness and equity.

Whereas before 1957 the death penalty had been mandatory for murder in England, Wales and Northern Ireland and also in Scotland, this had long ceased to be the case in the United States where gradually in state after state discretionary capital laws had replaced mandatory ones, even in states which distinguished between degrees of murder.[55] The reason for the growth of jury discretion over sentencing seems to have been partly a fear that juries would otherwise, in many cases, refuse to convict and partly a dislike and distrust of the use of executive power to commute capital sentences.[56] However, the granting of this responsibility to juries led, it was alleged, to the arbitrary and discriminatory exercise of their power of discretion to decide whether or not a convicted person should be executed.

In *Furman v. Georgia*, the Supreme Court ruled that the death penalty, when imposed by trial juries free to sentence a convicted person to death or alternatively to a lesser sentence without any standards or guidelines to assist or compel them to make rational and equitable choices, was "cruel and unusual punishment in violation of the Eighth and Fourteenth Amendments"[57] to the U.S. Constitution. The death penalty statutes that gave juries discretion over sentencing, which had been upheld only the previous year in *McGautha v. California*, were now held by a majority of five to four to be cruel and unusual and thus a denial of the due process of law guaranteed by the Fourteenth Amendment.[58] Two judges ruled that the death penalty was *per se* unconstitutional and three that the existing statutory jury discretion was unstructured and arbitrarily imposed and thus a denial of basic constitutional rights. Justice Stewart commented: "These death sentences are cruel and unusual in the same way that being struck by lightning is cruel and unusual…the petitioners are among a capriciously-selected random handful upon whom the sentence of death has in fact been imposed…I simply conclude that the Eighth and Fourteenth Amendments cannot tolerate the infliction of a sentence of death under legal systems that permit this unique penalty to be so wantonly and freakishly imposed."[59] Justice White noted that "there is no meaningful basis for distinguishing the few cases in which (capital punishment) is imposed from the many cases in which it is not.[60]

In the early part of the 20th century the American murder/execution ratio was estimated at between 70:1 and 85:1, but by the 1960s, it had risen to 504:1 and even the murder/death sentence ratio was 92:1, so that less than one person in five sentenced to death was executed. This may be contrasted with the figures for England and Wales 1900–1949 when the murder/execution ratio was 12:1 and just over a half of the persons sentenced to death were executed. Even when the much higher murder rate in the U.S.A. is allowed for (of the order of 20,000 per annum or 15 per 100,000 of population, compared with a total for England and Wales over the entire 50-year period 1900–1949 of about 7,500 or one-third of a murder per annum per 100,000 population), the proportion of murderers and even of those condemned to death who were finally executed is very low.[61] It is this fact that led the Supreme Court to call capital punishment an unusual punishment and when viewed in combination with the severity of death relative to other penalties an unconstitutionally "cruel and unusual punishment."

In 1972 Justice Douglas saw the death penalty as being applied not merely in a freakish but in a discriminatory way:

> The discretion of judges and juries in imposing the death penalty to be selectively applied, feeding prejudices against the accused if he is poor and despised and lacking political clout or if he is a member of a suspect or unpopular minority[62].... The death sentence is disproportionately imposed and carried out on the poor, the Negro and the members of unpopular groups.[63]

In consequence, he held that the death penalty as then administered was unconstitutional since it violated a convicted person's right to the equal protection of the laws even where the relevant statutes were nondiscriminatory.

After *Furman v. Georgia*, those who wanted to retain capital punishment were trapped in a cleft stick. Fully discretionary death sentences had been declared unconstitutional but so had mandatory death sentences as a result of the Supreme Court ruling in *McGautha v. California*. Nevertheless, after *Furman v. Georgia*, several states did enact mandatory death sentence laws which were then struck down by the Court as unconstitutional [*Woodson v. North Carolina* (1976), *Roberts (Stanislaus) v. Louisiana* (1977), *Lockett v. Ohio* (1978), *Bell v. Ohio* (1978)], again because they resulted in unfairness and were contrary to the rule of law and to due process. The reasoning behind this view is that the offender cannot have a fair trial if the sentencing court cannot or does not take into account all the relevant aggravating and mitigating factors. Implicitly, it is assumed here that the reason for having capital punishment is a moralist one, i.e., a mandatory penalty would result in the execution of some people whose degree of *guilt* was not sufficient to justify executing them. Also the Courts have held that a mandatory death penalty does not remove arbitrariness. It simply shifts it to another point in the system as juries refuse to convict in cases where they think the death penalty excessive or inappropriate.

Thus, any state that wished to restore capital punishment now had to steer a narrow course between unconstitutional "unguided discretion" and equally unconstitutional "no discretion" to arrive at an acceptable scheme of structured discretion since the Court had ruled that "discretion must be suitably directed and limited so as to minimize the risk of wholly arbitrary and capricious action."[64] The Supreme Court both here and indeed elsewhere, when striking down the death penalty for rape and other crimes not resulting in the death of the victim,[65] was guided by the moralist principle that no offender should be punished more than he or she deserves. Also, the Court took the view that no offender should be punished more than another offender whose offense and history revealed a similar pattern of aggravating and mitigating factors.

The Supreme Court has not abolished capital punishment in the United States and executions began again in 1977 after a 10-year moratorium, while the constitutional issues were being decided. However, the procedural rules are now so strict and the grounds (and opportunities) for appeal so numerous, various and complex that a murderer can only be executed after extremely costly, time-consuming, exhaustive and exhausting legal proceedings. It would be cheaper actually to keep a convicted murderer in jail for life than to negotiate such a Constitutional minefield.[66] The legal impediments to execution are such that capital punishment has been whittled away.

The Supreme Court consistently has shown a reluctance to try to resolve the kinds of causalist arguments about deterrence that dominated the debates within the British Parliament and to a lesser but still significant extent American political discourse. With the exception of Justice Marshall, the Supreme Court justices have not been willing to make a decision about the evidence for and against deterrence, but in *Gregg v. Georgia* (1976), Justice Stewart (joined by Justices Powell and Stevens) outlined many of the causalist arguments used in the British Parliament in 1957 and indeed again in 1983.[67] However, the responsibility for deciding this causalist factual issue was firmly handed to the State legislatures. Justice Stewart went on to comment:

> The value of capital punishment as a deterrent of crime is a complex factual issue the resolution of which lies with the legislature, which can evaluate the results of statistical studies in terms of their own local conditions and with a flexibility of approach that is not available to the courts.[68]

Chief Justice Burger, dissenting in *Furman v. Georgia* likewise had said:

> The case against capital punishment is not the product of legal dialectic but rests primarily on factual claims, the truth of which cannot be tested by conventional judicial processes.[69]

The Supreme Court's refusal to deal in detail with causalist arguments is an expression of the political doctrine of the division of power which assigns the political responsibility for lawmaking to the legislatures and is a refusal on the part of the Court to claim a legitimate and overriding expertise in areas other than constitutional law. The Supreme Court has said that the causalist case *against* deterrence is not sufficiently strong to make the Court rule that the death penalty is inevitably a cruel and unusual punishment unjustified by any legitimate social purpose, but that is all. If the Supreme Court had expressed a stronger view than this, either in support of the validity of the deterrence argument or against it, this might well have been an unconstitutional usurpation of the constitutional powers of the state legislatures.

Many American states now have produced new and, in some cases, constitutionally acceptable rules for the conduct of trials that can result in the imposition of the death penalty. These seem to be the product of the legislatures' causalist search for deterrence and the Supreme Court's moralist insistence on equity which operates as a retribution-based brake on the exercise of capital punishment. The calculations of American econometricians (if true, and this is an unresolved controversy) purport to show that in aggregate the lives of "x" victims are saved for every murderer that is executed,[70] but they can cast no light on the question of which individuals should be executed in order to maximize this deterrent effect. It is unlikely that the level of executions of America will ever come anywhere near the number of murders committed every year (of the order of 20,000),[71] or even that all murderers of a particular type (defined along the causalist lines of Britain's 1957 Homicide Act) could or would be executed. Only *some* of those who have committed "deterrable" murders will be sentenced to death and the only way in which these can be selected in order to avoid charges of arbitrariness or discrimination is in terms of moral culpability. In the long run, the tension between these disparate causalist and moralist forces probably will frustrate efforts to retain capital punishment in the United States.

The Future of the Controversies Over Capital Punishment and Abortion

A number of American political scientists have suggested that the transformation of contentious moral issues about life and death into more sober questions of constitutional law by transferring them from the political arena to the more detached Olympian world of the Supreme Court defuses potentially divisive problems.[72] However, in Western Europe, capital punishment has been abolished and abortion legalized by legislative action, and there has been less bitter controversy than in the United States. In Britain, there have been several attempts in the 1970's and 1980's to restore capital punishment or to restrict abortion by Private Members' legislation, but they all have failed and the new causalist status quo is reasonably stable.[73] Feminist pressure to make abortion on demand a woman's right likewise has lacked political clout, and the ineffectiveness of feminist resistance to changes in the time limit after which abortion may not be carried out[74] has revealed the impotence of the women's movement in Britain.

By contrast, in the United States capital punishment is still a controversial and divisive issue, even though the actual number of people being executed is very small. The dramatic protracted legal battles that take place before each execution serve only to polarize Americans into the camps of "law and order" and "crusading abolitionists" respectively. Similarly, the Supreme Court's 1973 rulings on abortion have, if anything, raised the temperature of the controversy. The anti-abortion lobby, having suffered a sudden and overwhelming defeat in the name of constitutional rights, will seek to amend the Constitution so as to grant rights to the fetus. Thus, the Supreme Court's attempt to resolve the abortion controversy by reference to the Constitution may provoke a battle over the wording and interpretation of American society's most fundamental moral document. The other tactics adopted by those who were outraged by the sudden demolition of restrictions on abortion, ranging from the Hyde Amendment [and the subsequent cases brought to the Supreme Court—*Beal v. Doe* (1977), *Maher v. Roe* (1977), *Harris v. McRae* (1980)][75] to the bombing of abortion clinics all indicate that abortion is still a far more contentious issue in the United States than it is in Britain and much of Western Europe. The reason probably lies in the greater strength in America of traditional religion-based morality, whether fundamentalist Protestant or Roman Catholic.

Why the Changes Took Place

In Western Europe, and especially Britain, and to a lesser but still significant extent, the United States, changes in the law relating to capital punishment and abortion have been part of a broad shift away from the traditional moralism of guilt and innocence towards a causalist ethic of minimizing harm. Causalism is the extension to private morality of an ethos which developed as a result of the growth of large institutions and the need to establish rules governing the relationships between them and between such institutions and individuals. Liability, regulation, insurance or welfare cannot be determined or administered on the basis of personal guilt or innocence. The key question that has to be asked in determining questions of legal liability is not "who is to blame?" but "who is to pay when things go wrong?"[76] A company has neither a body to be kicked nor a soul to be damned, but it does have a cash-box from which compensation may be paid and on which fines may be levied, even in cases where no one has deliberately or even negligently committed any transgression. If personal guilt had to be proven in each case, much regulatory legislation would break down or become impossibly costly to police. Insurance is not merely a system of risk-spreading but also one of guilt- and blame-spreading. The damage caused by the sins of the drunken driver, the negligent surgeon, the arsonist, the glutton, is paid for out of the increased premiums paid by the virtuous and lucky. The difficulty and expense of disentangling bad luck, negligence and wickedness is such that insurance companies often do not bother to probe questions of culpability at all. State welfare is administered on a universal and bureaucratic basis with little attempt to discriminate between the deserving and the undeserving poor, between the unfortunate and the feckless. When old-age pensions were first introduced in Britain in the early years of the 20th century, there was strong pressure to grant them only to those who had led respectable lives and to withhold them from those with a history of unrepentant wickedness. It was impossible to do so and today we are amazed that such a scheme could even have been suggested. Likewise, it is difficult for outsiders to sympathize with the view of the former Irish Prime Minister, Mr. Haughey, that habitual criminals should be denied legal aid for their defense on the grounds that they don't deserve it.[77]

Today, it is often the innocent victim who is penalized, the guilty person who is assisted, simply because, from the state's point of view it is a more effective way of minimizing harm. In West Germany, it is an offense to leave a car unlocked because it might get stolen, and in Britain, diabetics are indignant because unregistered drug addicts (i.e., who buy on the black market) are given free, fresh clean syringes and needles, whereas the diabetics have to pay. Diabetics are careful injectors, but addicts are not, and the clean needles are issued to try to stop the spread of tetanus, hepatitis and AIDS among addicts by the use of unclean shared needles. The causalist bureaucrat is not concerned with whether people get their just deserts, merely with minimizing harm.

The changes in the way those with the power to implement morality have come to perceive issues such as capital punishment or abortion is the most recent stage in the spread of causalist morality. Other indirect but, in some ways, more far-reaching decisions about life and death such as safety regulations, laws regarding the hygienic preparation of food, compulsory third-party motor insurance, the chlorination and fluoridation of water supplies and the establishment of smokeless zones, have since been decided on a causalist basis. Abortion and capital punishment have now also been brought under the causalist umbrella. In a causalist society, the strongest moral imperative is the avoidance of harm, pain or suffering of all kinds. Retribution, corporal punishments, penance and mortification of the flesh have no place in a causalist world and the person in pain who refuses the effective chemical easements afforded by modern anesthetics, analgesics, or antidepressants, is not an admired stoic but an eccentric clown. Attempted suicides are treated with sympathy (and have increased in consequence)[78] and successful suicides are pitied, not condemned. Those who could no longer bear their suffering are no longer tipped without ceremony into a grave dug at a crossroads at midnight but buried with respect and even honor. For the causalist, the bans on divorce, contraception or abortion imposed by traditional moralists are not merely meaningless but evil because they cause pain to particular thwarted individuals and thus offend against the central principle of causalist morality. For the causalist, suffering is always an unmitigated evil and traditional moralist views of the virtues of stoical self-sacrifice, of willingness to endure and transcend one's allotted afflictions, of spiritual growth and redemption through the acceptance of suffering are repulsive nonsense. The causalist is stirred to righteous rage by the very existence of moralist rules that are seen as trapping individuals into a fatalistic acceptance of avoidable suffering. The response of causalists to situations of this kind shows that their ethic is not just an administrative calculus, but can be a strongly held moral creed. For the causalist, the woman at risk who has undergone amniocentesis and chosen to abort a fetus diagnosed as severely, genetically defective on the basis of chromosome analysis, is a rational and moral person. Those who would try to obstruct her are reprehensible men who are willing to inflect immeasurable suffering on the woman and her family in the name of the meaningless principle drawn from an alien and anachronistic rival moral system. If the moralists should compound their wickedness by praising the struggles and sacrifices of women and families that have patiently accepted such an affliction, the causalist will see them as liars and humbugs into the bargain. The moralists' refusal to contemplate the abortion of, say, a fetus known to be afflicted with Tay-Sachs disease[79] is as monstrously wicked for the causalist as abortion on demand is for the traditional moralist. At this personal level, the causalists' most strongly held moral view is that no one should be expected to put up with major avoidable suffering. Once again, it is clear that moralists and causalists differ so much in their central moral assumptions that they will have difficulty in understanding and sympathizing with one another's arguments and passions.

The process of change in Britain is a typical case of the rise of the causalist ethic and the experience of much of Western Europe is rather similar. In America, however, moralisms are stronger because of the way they define both the basic national identity of the country and the identity of the various unmelted ethnics. In the homogeneous long-established nation states of Western Europe, identity is relatively unproblematic and sufficiently defined by geography or language. The United States, by contrast, is both a new nation and a nation of immigrants. For the nation as a whole, the Constitution is a statement of what it is to be an American, a vital component of America's civic religion, the American way of life. At a more local level, identity, ethnicity and community are expressed through religious denominations which have far more regular adherents than is the case in most European countries.[80] In consequence, Roman Catholicism and fundamentalist Protestantism have more grassroot and political strength in America than in any other Western country, except the two Irelands (where ethnicity and religion reinforce each other even more strongly). Creeping secularization has affected America like other Western countries and ethos of American institutions is often as causalist as it is elsewhere. However, the more illiberal denominations still have the power to fight hard against particular moral shifts that pose a symbolic threat to their world view, such as the abolition of capital punishment or freely available abortion. Faced with the successful use of blocking tactics in the dispersed legislatures of this more plural society, the reformers have appealed to the secular defining rules for American society as a whole—to the rights guaranteed by the Constitution.

NOTES

1. In order to reduce the number of variables involved, I have in general restricted myself to a consideration of the changes taking place in those capitalist democracies with a predominantly European cultural tradition, i.e., the United States, Western Europe and the old Commonwealth.

2. These dates are somewhat arbitrary since in some cases capital punishment was suspended before being abolished and in others the state retains the right to execute people in wartime or for military offenses—treason or piracy. See Amnesty International (1979). The death penalty was effectively abolished even earlier in the Scandinavian countries, Italy, West Germany, the Netherlands and Portugal. In Australia, the individual states of the Commonwealth have their own legislation, but the death penalty has been abolished in Queensland (1921), Tasmania (1968), Victoria (1975) and also, to all intents and purposes, in New South Wales (1955).

3. Compiled on the basis of data in Bedau (ed).

4. See Loraine, 163–165 and Jaffe *et.al.* (eds.) 2–3.

5. Based on data from Institut National d'Études Démographiques [referred to henceforth as INED] and Potts and Selman.

6. In the Netherlands, the law is simply not enforced. English-Welsh laws prohibiting abortion never extended to Scotland, which has its own legal system and local customary restrictions simply withered away. See INED 19, 29, 47–48.

7. See INED 11, 25–6, 29–30, 47.

8. INED 19.

9. For a detailed discussion, see Davies (1975), "How Our Rulers Argue about Censorship," in Dhavan and Davies (eds); Davies, "Moralists, Causalists, Sex, Law and Morality" in W. H. G. Armytage, R. Chester, and John Peel (eds.).

10. See Hansard, vol. 732, col. 1067, 1075 and 1154, and Hansard, vol. 750, col. 1347–1348.

11. See P. G. Richards, 97.

12. See INED, 123–124, Medical Protection Society, 99–110, and Walbert and Butler, 329–330.

13. See Hansard, vol. 750, col. 1180–1181.

14. Simms and Hindel, 70.

15. Hansard, vol. 750, col. 1175.

16. Hansard, vol. 750, col.1165–1166. See also cols. 1176–1177.

17. There may well be a difference. See Luker, 18–39, Mohr, Rubin, 14, and Sarvis and Rodman, 18–19.

18. See Rubin, 20–22, Sarvis and Rodman, 63–64.

19. See Jaffe *et. al.*, 4.

20. Personal observation by the author who was in Italy at the time. See also Berlinguer, 23–25, and comments by Drs. Falanga and F. D'Ippolito in INED, 95–96.
21. See Luker, 73–74.
22. See INED 148, for a summary and also 63, 129–130, 132–133, 141–147.
23. See Sarvis and Rodman, 30–33.
24. See Sarvis and Rodman, 40–41, and *Model Penal Code*, American Law Institute 1962, 189–190.
25. See Brandon and Davies and see Bedau, 234–240.
26. This is true in the short term *but* there seems to also have been earlier patterns of change that are difficult to analyze. See Tuttle, 48, 102, and Meltsner, 50.
27. See Tuttle, 71–72 and 118–119.
28. E.g., see Hansard, vol. 449, cols.1014, 1030, 1053–1054, 1067–1070.
29. E.g., see Hansard, vol. 449, cols. 1014 and 1035.
30. Amnesty International, 120–121.
31. Amnesty International, 117.
32. Amnesty 104, 111, 121. This, of course, leaves open the interesting question of why these countries had abolished capital punishment in the first place at an earlier time [Denmark 1930, Iceland 1928, Netherlands 1870, Norway 1905, Sweden 1921] than is the case for those discussed on p. 102 and whether they did so for moralist or causalist reasons. The small Benelux and Scandinavian countries were at the time when they abolished capital punishment, all very unviolent places, not only internally but *also* in their external relations where they were all neutral *pays fainéants*. In such countries, the moralist forces upholding capital punishment are likely to be weak. See Davies in Badham (ed.), "Religion, State, and Society" Mellen, 1989.
33. See Amnesty International, 104, 108, 111, 175–176.
34. See Royal Commission.
35. See Royal Commission, 17–18.
36. See Royal Commission, 158–162 and 206–207 and Bedau, 4–6.
37. See Bedau, 279.
38. I have deliberately taken a "moralist" phrase from the comments attached to the American Law Institute's *Model Penal Code* (draft No. 9, 1959), 71. See Bedau, 279.
39. See Tuttle, 128.
40. Hansard, vol. 704, col. 908.
41. See Hansard, July 13, 1983, vol. 45, Issue 1283, cols. 892–996, and Davies, "Britain Debates the Morality (or Utility) of the Rope," *Wall Street Journal*, July 13, 1983, and *The Times*, July 14, 1983, 4.
42. Hansard, vol. 732, col. 1101. See also vol. 750, col. 1353.
43. See Bedau, 102, 248 and 305–307, and see James Q. Wilson, 206, *et. seq.*
44. E.g., see Laurence R. Klein, Brian Forst and Victor Filato, "The Deterrent

Effect of Capital Punishment—An Assessment of the Evidence" in Bedau, 138–158, and Hans Zeisel, "The Deterrent Effect of the Death Penalty: Facts v. Faith," in Bedau, 117–137.

45. American patterns of belief and commitment are in many ways as secularized as those of Western Europe, though religiosity and rates of participation are far higher. See Wilson, 109–113, and Herberg, 79, 80, 92, 271. I would add, however, that the zeal is for real.

46. See Sarkis and Rodman, 141–142, Luker, 69–90.

47. See Bedau, 22, *et. seq.*, Sarkis and Rodman, 66–67.

48. See Christoph, 153–155.

49. See *Roe v. Wade* and Walbert and Butler, 349–350.

50. See *Roe v. Wade*, Section 8, Sarkis and Rodman, 64, Walbert and Butler, 340.

51. John Locke quoted in Rubin, 78.

52. See *Roe v. Wade.*

53. See comment in Rubin, 71.

54. See *Roe v. Wade*, Leiser, 38–40. Sarkis and Rodman, 65.

55. See Bedau, 10–11.

56. See Bedau, 10 and Royal Commission, 206.

57. See also Pannick, 96.

58. See also Pannick, 95 and 102–103.

59. *Furman* 33 L.Ed 2d, 390. See also Pannick, 96.

60. *Furman* 33 L.Ed 2d, 392. See also Pannick, 96.

61. Based on data from Bedau, 30–31, and Royal Commission, 326–327 and 334–335.

62. *Furman v. Georgia* 33 L.Ed 2d, 358.

63. *Furman v. Georgia* 33 L.Ed 2d, 355. Justice Douglas is quoting from *"The Challenge of Crime in a Free Society,"* the Report of the President's Commission on Law Enforcement and Administration of Justice, 1967.

64. See *Gregg v. Georgia.* See also Pannick, 97.

65. See *Coker v. Georgia* and also Pannick, 140.

66. See Barry Nakell, *The Cost of the Death Penalty*, in Bedau, 241–246, and also the comment by Justice Marshall in *Furman v. Georgia* 33 P.Ed 2d, 417.

67. See *Gregg v. Georgia* 50 P.Ed. 2d, 881–882.

68. *Gregg v. Georgia* 50 P.Ed 2d, 882. See also Pannick, 42–43 and 63.

69. *Furman v. Georgia* 33 P.Ed 2d 405. See also Pannick, 66.

70. E.g., see Isaac Ehrlich, "The Deterrent Effect of Capital Punishment: A Question of Life and Death," *American Economic Review*, vol. 68, June 1975. 397–417. J. A. Yunker. "Is the Death Penalty a Deterrent to Homicide? Some Time Series Evidence," *Journal of Behavioural Economics*, vol. 5, 1976, 45–81. David P. Phillips, "The Deterrent Effect of Capital Punishment, New Evidence on an Old Controversy," *American Journal of Sociology*, vol. 86, 1980, 139–148.

71. See *FBI Uniform Crime Reports*, 1978, 46, 57, 83.

72. See Rubin, 170.
73. See D. Marsh and D. Chambers, "The Abortion Lobby: Pluralism At Work" in Marsh (ed.), 144–165.
74. See Davies, 1988, Britain: "Abortion Debate Obscures Issues," *Wall Street Journal,* February 17th.
75. See also Jaffe *et.al.,* 127–140.
76. See Davies, 1975, 207–210 and Lord Devlin, *The Enforcement of Morals,* London, Oxford U.P. 1965, 27–34.
77. See Dáil Debates, vol. 193, cols. 234–235, 15 February 1962. Mr. Haughey was then Minister of Justice. See also Claire P. Carney, "The Growth of Legal Aid in the Republic of Ireland," *The Irish Jurist* New Series, vol. 14, 1979, 61–82 and 211–228. Regarding the strength of anti-abortion moralism in Eire, see Rynne.
78. See Jean Baechler, *Suicides,* Oxford Basil Blackwell, 1979, 402–403. Baechler's data and analysis present a serious problem for the causalist for he has uncovered what amounts to a serious flaw in the causalists' argument even when viewed from within their own moral framework.
79. See comments in Jaffe *et. al.,* 157 and in M. Neil Macintyre, *Genetic Risk, Prenatal Diagnosis and Selective Abortion,* in Walbert and Butler (eds.).
80. See Herburg, 10–13.

SELECT BIBLIOGRAPHY

Amnesty International, *The Death Penalty,* (London: Amnesty International, 1979).

W.H.G. Armytage, R. Chester and John Peel (eds.), *Changing Patterns of Sexual Behaviour,* (London: Academic Press, 1980).

Hugo Adam Bedau (ed.), *The Death Penalty in America,* 3rd ed. (New York: Oxford University Press, 1983).

Giovanni Berlinguer, *La Legge Sull' Aborto,* (Rome: Riunite, 1978).

Ruth Brandon and Christie Davies, *Wrongful Imprisonment, Mistaken Convictions and Their Consequences* (London: Allen and Unwin, 1973).

E. Roy Calvert, *Capital Punishment in the 20th Century,* 5th ed. (London: Putnam, 1936).

James B. Christoph, *Capital Punishment and British Politics* (London: Allen and Unwin, 1962).

Church Assembly Board for Social Responsibility, *Abortion, An Ethical Discussion* (London: Church Information Office, 1965).

Christie Davies, *Permissive Britain, Social Change in the Sixties and Seventies* (London: Pitman, 1975).

Rajeev Dhavan and Christie Davies (eds.), *Censorship and Obscenity* (London: Martin Robertson, 1978).

Fred M. Frohock, *Abortion, A Case Study in Law and Morals* (Westport, Connecticut: Greenwood, 1983).

Will Herberg, *Protestant, Catholic, Jew* (Garden City, New York: Doubleday, 1960).

William Bradford Huie, *The Execution of Private Slovik* (New York: New American Library, 1954).

Institute National d'Etudes Démographiques (INED), *L'interruption volontaire de grosseuse dans l'Europe des neuf (Cahier No.91)* (Paris: Presses Universitaires de France, 1981).

Frederick S. Jaffe, Barbara L. Lindheim, and Philip R. Lee, *Abortion Politics, Private Morality and Public Policy* (New York: McGraw-Hill, 1981).

Burton M. Leiser (ed.), *Values in Conflict Life, Liberty and the Rule of Law* (New York: Macmillan, 1981).

John A. Loraine, *Syndromes of the Seventies Population, Sex and Social Change* (London: Peter Owen, 1978).

Kristin Luker, *Abortion and the Politics of Motherhood* (Berkeley: University of California Press, 1984).

David Marsh (ed.), *Pressure Politics, Interest Groups in Britain* (London: Junction, 1983).

The Medical Protection Society, *The Abortion Act 1967: Proceedings of a Symposium* (London: Pitman, 1969).

Michael Meltsner, *Cruel and Unusual, The Supreme Court and Capital Punishment* (New York: Random House, 1973).

James C. Mohr, *Abortion in America: The Origins and Evolution of National Policy* (New York: Oxford University Press, 1978).

David Pannick, *Judicial Review of the Death Penalty* (London: Duckworth, 1982).

Malcolm Potts and Peter Selman, *Society and Fertility* (Plymouth: Macdonald and Evans, 1979).

Peter G. Richards, *Parliament and Conscience* (London: Allen and Unwin, 1970).

Royal Commission on Capital Punishment 1949–1953, *Report* (Cmd.) 8932 (London: H.M.S.O., 1953).

Eva R. Rubin, *Abortion, Politics and the Courts, Roe v. Wade and its Aftermath* (Westport, Connecticut: Greenwood).

Andrew Rynne, *Abortion, the Irish Question* (Dublin: Ward River, 1982).

Betty Sarvis and Hyman Rodman, *The Abortion Controversy* (New York: Columbia University Press, 1974).

Madelaine Simms and Keith Hindell *Abortion Law Reformed* (London: Peter Owen, 1971).

Elizabeth Orman Tuttle, *The Crusade Against Capital Punishment in Great Britain* (London: Stevens, 1961).

David F. Walbert and J. Douglas Butler (eds.), *Abortion, Society and the Law* (Cleveland: Case Western Reserve Press, 1973).

Bryan Wilson, *Religion in Secular Society* (Harmondsworth: Penguin, 1969).

James Q. Wilson, *Thinking About Crime* (New York: Basic, 1975 and 1983).

British Parliamentary Debates

All references to "Hansard" refer to Hansard Official Reports of Parliamentary Debates 5th Series House of Commons.

Selected American Supreme Court Cases

Beal v. Doe (1977) 432 US 438; 97 S Ct 2366; 53 L.Ed 2d, 464

Bell v. Ohio (1978) 428 US 909; 98 S Ct 2977; 57 L.Ed 2d, 797

Coker v. Georgia (1977) 433 US 485; 97 S Ct 2861; 53 L.Ed 2d, 982

Doe v. Bolton (1973) 410 US 179; 93 S Ct 739; 35 L.Ed 2d, 201

Furman v. Georgia (1972) 408 US 238; 92 S Ct 2726; 33 L.Ed 2d, 346

Gregg v. Georgia (1976) 428 US 153; 96 S Ct 3235; 50 L.Ed 2d, 30

Harris v. McFae (1980) 448 US 297; 100 S Ct 2671; 65 L.Ed 2d, 784

Lockett v. Ohio (1978) 438 US 586; 98 S Ct 2954; 57 L.Ed 2d, 973

Maher v. Doe (1977) 432 US 526; 97 S Ct 2474; 53 L.Ed 2d, 534

McGautha v. California (1971) 402 US 183; 91 S Ct 1454; 28 L.Ed 2d, 711

Roberts (Harry) v. Louisiana (1977) 431 US 633; 97 S Ct 1993; 52 L.Ed 2d, 188

Roberts (Stanislaus) v. Louisiana (1976) 428 US 325; 96 S Ct 3001; 49 L.Ed 2d, 974

Roe v. Wade (1973) 410 US 113; 93 S Ct 705; 35 L.Ed 2d, 147

Woodson v. North Carolina (1976) 428 US 280; 96 S Ct 2978; 49 L.Ed 2d, 944

<u>SEVEN</u>

"WANTED" and "UNWANTED" LIFE

THE IMPACT OF NEW SCIENCE ON ETHICS, LAW AND PUBLIC POLICY

Nicholas Kittrie

Introduction: The Determination of Value

The development of advanced and highly sophisticated biomedical technologies presents new and complex questions for those concerned with matters of human life—be they in medicine, or the biological sciences or in the clergy, law, or other policy disciplines. This paper examines a number of areas in which biomedical advancements are likely to influence the way we consider and attempt to resolve issues of life and death.

Our analysis emphasizes questions concerning the life-enhancing process rather than the issues relating to the termination of life. It should be noted, moreover, that it is the ethical, legal and public policy implications of these biomedical developments, rather than their underlying scientific bases, that we will explore and discuss. This emphasis is due to the fact that the writer is better versed in the jurisprudential and policy disciplines that relate to "values" than the scientific disciplines which directly affect the management and manipulation of life and death. Furthermore, in surveying the growing number of legal and policy issues, we will not attempt a comprehensive resolution of the questions raised, because no paper as brief as this one can adequately come to grips with the topic, nor will any hasty set of answers satisfy the needs of this complex arena. It is hoped, however, that this paper will stimulate greater future attention to the "values" dilemmas clustered around the life-enhancing processes.

To avoid abruptly entering the specific problem area explored in this paper (that of the preserving, extension, and initiation of human life), several precautionary observations need to be made regarding this committee's overall task to explore "the value of human life." Value is an undefined term with potentially broad meanings and implications. In considering value, both the type of disciplinary scales utilized and the perspective of the weighmaster must be evaluated. One may weigh value by using economic, social, political, moral, or religious scales. A human life which may claim little economic value may, nevertheless, possess great religious value. Likewise, a life with marginal moral value (e.g., that of an unscrupulous dictator) may loom high in the political arena. Great sensitivity and constant awareness are, therefore, required to balance the diverse and often contradictory weights attributed to any given life by the differing disciplines.

Equally, attention must be directed to the diverse perspectives from which the value of human life can be viewed. The measurement of value greatly depends on the weighmaster's perspective. One may dramatize the variety of perspectives by asking: "value to whom?" Is value to be measured from the perspective of the individual whose life is under consideration, the perspective of his family (wife, children, parents), or should a broader perspective of "society" or "state" be utilized for measurement? Again, one readily discovers that what may be considered a valuable life by the principal may be perceived as an undue hardship by the family. At times the reverse may be true: a life discarded by the principal may be heroically upheld by the family. Finally, a life viewed as unworthy of living by a principal, his family, or both, might often, nonetheless, represent value to society, the state, or the public interest—hence, the traditional laws which prohibit voluntary as well as involuntary euthanasia.

In structuring a fair and socially acceptable process for decision-making regarding issues of human value, one must, therefore, be constantly cognizant not only of the competing disciplinary points of view, but also the diverse perspectives which need to be considered and weighed. How much attention should be given to the viewpoint of the elderly and chronically disabled principal who seeks to go on living despite a previously difficult life? Should one accept and rely upon the judgment of a young but depressed family member for whom living has lost, possibly temporarily, all value? Should psychiatric testimony or religious values be solicited? Should one listen instead to the wishes of a family or community long exhausted by the burdens and costs of maintaining life for one of its members? And what if the scene is diametrically reversed: a loving and committed family seeking to preserve and lengthen the life of an unwilling or unconscious member?

The judgmental relativism with regard to the value of human life, produced by the different disciplinary viewpoints and perspectives, is further heightened by the historical, as well as, contemporary debate on the commencement and termination of human life. "When does life begin and when does it end?" For much of society the answer is to be found in positive law—in the products of the legislative or judicial branches. Yet, these laws and decisions are mostly transitory. To some the ultimate answer is to be found in science, yet science has not been able or willing to yield an unambiguous response. Others proclaim that life and death belong to the realm of religion and belief and that absolute answers are to be found in the fundamental doctrines of one faith or another.

In the United States, the Supreme Court has entered the breach on several occasions in an effort to narrow the conflict between science, religion, public policy, and individual privacy. Seeking to breach the conflicts, the Court articulated legal doctrines in an effort to shape practical public policy solutions. Yet, in its proposed solutions, the Court has left unanswered the precise timing of either life or death, preferring instead to base its judgment on the constitutional concept of the "persons." This term, as the Court concluded approvingly, has been reserved traditionally to a live post-birth human being, thus leaving the unborn fetus outside the realm of the constitution's due process and other protections of the person. *Roe v. Wade*, 410 U.S. 113 (1973). Even with this cautious and narrow approach, the United States Supreme Court readily discovered that one cannot even so slightly enter the marketplace of "human life" definitions without being tarred and bruised. While this paper will refrain from venturing further into this definitional morass, the reader must once more be alerted to the relativistic and shifting undercurrents which endanger any effort to reasonably discuss and assess, not only the value of human life, but also the time of its commencement and conclusion.

Pro-Life and Pro-Quality of Life

Although widely disparate in their views, those speaking out on issues of human life may be divided, for the most part, into two camps. What separates the two are their philosophical or axiomatic premises.

The first group views life as a divine gift endowed with divine qualities. These divine dimensions may not be interfered with by profane and man-made devices, priorities or schemes. Human life is holy and anything in the whole world that contains either realized life or a potential glimmer of life may not be infringed upon for any reason. Members of this group are likely to profess a fundamental opposition to any interference by individuals or society with the sanctity of human life, whether in the form of birth control, abortion or euthanasia.

The second group considers life not as a divine gift, but as a worldly and aesthetic experience. To this group, what matters most is not life *per se*, but the quality of life—with an emphasis on the good life. Accordingly, this group might accept societal planning and intervention because it views society's total well-being as more important than attention to and the preservation of each individual life.

It may not be unfair to label the first category of scientists, thinkers and policy formulators as adherents of the "Pro-Sanctity of Life" view, or briefly *"Pro-Lifers."* In their view, life needs to be preserved at any cost, whether individual or social. The second category might be tagged, again not unfairly, as the "Pro-Quality of Life" camp. To this group, considerations of the overall or holistic individual welfare, as well as the overall societal good, are the controlling goals. It is not life as such that should be guarded and preserved, but the good life, and that for the greatest number of potential beneficiaries. Surprisingly, however, the two camps tend to reverse their positions with regard to capital punishment, a practice more generally supported by the conservative pro-lifers than by the more liberal adherents of the quality of life.

Reviewing the "human life" literature, whether scientific or policy-oriented, developing during the post-World War II era, one readily discerns that only a small segment of practitioners and ethicists has concerned itself primarily with questions revolving around the preserving, securing, extending or even initiating of human life. The larger group has concentrated, instead, on problems and practices relating to the shortening or termination of existing human life, as well as the prevention of the potentially undesirable life.

As one examines the papers prepared for this committee, one notes the predominance of topics on the extinguishment of life, to which the pro-lifers are most sensitive. These topics, including abortion, birth control and the right to die (euthanasia), are central pillars in the programs of the quality of life camp but constitute fighting words for those committed to pro-life. Only two of the papers presented before the committee dwell not on the shortening, termination or prevention of human life, but on other issues which can be viewed more neutrally by both the pro-lifers and the pro-quality of life communities. These are the paper on the "Moral Implications of the Manipulations of the Genetic Nature of Man" and the paper on "Searching For a New Life Style."

In contrast with this general trend, our essay's major effort is to direct the attention of this committee and the readers to a host of the topics clustering around the creation and extension of human life, rather than those dealing with life termination. This essay, after some preliminary observations, steers clear of those issues concerning the value of human life that are currently in the midst of hot debates—including the questions of birth control, abortion and euthanasia. In these latter arenas, the conflict lines between pro-life and pro-quality of life advocates have been clearly drawn; the war is on, and no truce is in sight.

Unwanted and Wanted Life

For the past three decades, the major debates in the human life arena have concentrated on issues of unwanted life. The specific issues have included: voluntary euthanasia, birth control, suspension of heroic medicine for those beyond recovery and abortion. In all the above instances, there usually exists a living and principal advocate for the termination or prevention of life. In the case of voluntary euthanasia, it is an aged or ill person seeking a peaceful expiration. In the case of birth control, the principal is often a sexually active individual advocating the use of sex as an instrument of recreation rather than procreation. In instances involving the suspension of heroic medicine, there is a family member or guardian seeking to stop the drain on family resources. And in the case of abortion, there is again the mother's desire to be relieved of the burdens of an unwanted pregnancy and parenthood.

Only in the area of birth control has society molded a relatively acceptable solution. Despite birth control's affinity to the pro-life agendas, most societies have recognized the distance between the prevention of conception and the termination of life or potential life. Thus, even though in Puritan and Victorian America birth control devices were frowned upon and even criminalized, there has been no substantial outcry against the judicial abolition of criminal sanctions against prophylactics. When the United States Supreme Court held in *Griswold v. Connecticut*, 381 U.S. 479 (1965), that the right of family privacy, which includes the procreation decision, took precedence over the general protection of public morality, which accounted for the prohibition of prophylactics, few individuals stood up in protest. No stronger was the opposition to the court's decision to extend this same right of privacy to unmarried couples. *Eisenstadt v. Baird*, 405 U.S. 438 (1972).

Yet, both the legal and public response to birth control issues has been unlike the response to the other three instances of unwanted life. Voluntary euthanasia continues to be treated as murder or suicide, regardless of the humane motives of the actor and only judicial sentencing discretion saves those engaging in the practice from severe statutorily enumerated sanctions. The suspension of heroic medicine, similarly, has not found its appropriate place of rest. Following the national drama which surrounded the Quinlan case in 1976 (*Matter of Quinlan,* 70 N.J. 10, 355 A. 2d 647), some of the hospital practices regarding comatose and brain-dead patients have been relaxed. There also has been a redefining, through legislation, of the medical definition of death to permit greater discretion to health practitioners in bringing to a conclusion a patient's dependence upon heroic medical procedures. The severe sanctions of criminal law remain, however, only in obeyance: for as long as a life continues to legally exist in a patient, no judge, physician, nor family member can authorize its execution without fear of criminal penalties. Placing the legal hazards aside, great debates still persist over the moral, religious and ethical issues raised by "brain-dead" termination cases. Even where criminal penalties do not apply, many families struggle with the emotional effect of such a decision.

With regard to abortion, likewise, a clear and permanent solution might not be at hand. Upholding the fetus' traditional exemption from the protections offered "persons" under the Constitution, American law now permits women, in the exercise of their privacy rights, to resort to an abortion, virtually at will, during the first trimester of pregnancy. *Roe v. Wade,* 410 U.S. 113 (1973). Only during the third trimester is the fetus' potential life recognized to the degree that individual states may either regulate abortion or altogether prohibit the practice. But even this carefully-tailored solution has had a rocky road since it was first articulated by the United States Supreme Court. Moreover, the future direction of the abortion laws cannot be readily foretold.

In the pages that follow, we will address a new and different range of life value issues which, despite their growing importance, have been greatly neglected. These issues involve not those who wish to die or cause death, prevent life or shorten it. Our agenda revolves around those who wish to live, to lengthen life or to create life. We will explore, as a consequence, the topics of heroic medicine, organ transplantation, artificial insemination and surrogate parenting. All these procedures, while fundamentally pro-life in their initial thrust, frequently seek to attain goals which strongly appeal also to those committed to the pro-quality of life persuasion.

Of primary concern to us will be the role of the new and advanced biomedical technology as a tool for life extension, for more effective mating, and possibly also as a vehicle for the attainment of the ancient goals of immortality or resurrection. Although detailed information, statistical data and cost figures for the increasing role of high-tech in the arena of human life might be lacking, the fundamental issues posed by high-tech can be readily outlined. They revolve, first, around the questions of cost, availability and the distribution of high-tech procedures and services. Second, high-tech poses a host of new moral and legal concerns resulting from the contemporary man's or woman's moving away from the traditional family-based operation to a non-familial and less-communal social environment.

Medical Science and Wanted Life

Leaving behind the moral, legal and policy questions posed by unwanted life to concentrate on issues related to wanted life, our first task is to define the meaning of "wanted life." For purposes of discussion, we will divide "wanted life" into two categories: (1) procedures for the continuation of an existing life, and (2) procedures for the creation of a new life. The former category, concerned with continuation or extension of existing life, we will designate as the "ongoing living" or "the willing to live" category. The latter category, which dwells not on the continuation but on the creation of new life, we will describe as "the new living" or the "willing to procreate" category.

In the arena of wanted life, the primary questions are not when and how a life or a potential life begins and when it may be extinguished, but when and how it may be extended or created. Because of its life-extending and life-improving proclivity, the wanted life arena appeared to be immune to the conflicts which have plagued the unwanted life territory. In the latter arena, as we have seen, the advocates of change and "reform," advancing mostly pro-quality of life arguments, have engaged in battle with the pro-lifers who have sought to maintain the status quo. In the area of wanted life, with its emphasis on pro-life procedures and pursuits, one should expect no similar confrontations.

Yet, even in the arena of "wanted life," pro-lifers and pro-quality of lifers might not be fully in agreement. Many pro-lifers, although advocating the preservation of unwanted life, find the scientifically innovative techniques for the creation of wanted life troublesome. The pro-lifers dilemma goes to illustrate that the public divisions regarding issues of life and death may not be truly dictated by pro-life and pro-quality of life doctrinal differences. The divisions might be derived, instead, from a fundamental break between those favoring scientific and social innovations and those in support of a more natural status quo.

Nevertheless, in the "wanted life" arena private and public passions, as yet, have not been fully aroused or inflamed. Public attention in this arena has dwelled more on the wonders of science and technology than on issues of morality, justice and public policy. But as innovative pro-life technology is becoming more prevalent and commonplace, the wonderment is bound to cease and inherent conflicts of interest and of values are likely to be manifested.

At its core, the wanted life arena does not involve any of the negative interventions with human life which are typical to the unwanted life category. Therefore, the traditional pro-life forces have not risen in alarm to protest against the innovative wanted life practices and procedures. But this is not to say that this arena is free of potential disagreement or strife. For there is in the new life-extending and life-creating technologies a sufficient departure from the usual courses of nature to create potentials, not only for economic conflicts, but also for philosophical, moral, and legal disagreements. These we set out to explore below.

The Willing to Live

Men, women and children of varying ages, who require the aid of organ transplants or other forms of heroic medicine for their continued living, are grouped under the "willing to live" category. By and large, this group consists of those who due to their legal age and mental capacity may be consulted with to determine their own wishes. We do not deal in these instances with a mentally undeveloped fetus whose wishes cannot be ascertained. The principal in this category is a living human being, a constitutionally defined "person" who is able to proclaim his pro-life choice. Nonetheless, that choice cannot always be freely exercised through private contractual pursuits. Those making a free pro-life election are often handicapped by either or both the economic costs and the scarcity of the resources required to implement their decision. The costs of heroic medicine, in many instances, are monumental. Indeed, several state governments have had to prohibit expensive organ transplants of Medicare patients in order to insure adequate funding for basic overall medical coverage. The availability of certain organs required for transplanting is in short supply. The demand for such transplants continues to increase and unfortunately the donor supply is not keeping pace. In 1986 alone, there were 8,000 kidney transplants performed, more than double the number of operations performed in 1981. Moreover, some 9,000 critical patients await donors and some 25,000 more potential beneficiaries require kidney transplants. [See, *Transplants, Who Lives, Who Dies,* Washington Post Health Sect., p. 12, col. 1, January 20, 1987.] As the biomedical technologies improve and expand, both costs and short supplies are going to make the question of beneficiary selection more difficult.

Is the allocation of these pro-living services to depend exclusively upon the material resources of the person in need? Should public resources be made available for this purpose and how should these resources be distributed? Should age and life expectancy constitute appropriate criteria? Should social utility, measured by one scale or another, be weighed in the process? Should such public priorities be the exclusive criteria in cases of extreme scarcity, granting the beneficiary's private resources no weight in the decision-making?

As one examines the host of economic, as well as ethical, questions relating to the heroic extension of an existing life, one cannot fail to recognize the connection between these questions and the ultimate meaning of the constitutionally protected "right to life." In the American legal tradition, the rights of life, liberty and property have been accorded special protection through both the Fifth and the Fourteenth Amendments to the United States Constitution. Designed primarily to guard against governmental encroachments without the benefits of "due process," these rights have been viewed primarily as negative, not positive, in character. Consequently, the right-to-life has been construed not as an entitlement but as a safeguard. In the face of the new medical technology, should the right-to-life be transformed, however, into a positive entitlement? Should such a transformation present an additional claim against the public treasury and resources? This, and related questions, has been troubling the medical community and the public at large for some time, but the fast-moving progress of science is likely to make them even more critical.

This is not the appropriate time or place for seeking a comprehensive answer to the questions of resources and scarcity, but some efforts in that direction might be desirable. At the very least, one should utilize this occasion to set out an agenda for future deliberations. This agenda must include the following questions: (1) Is there now or should there be a public duty to supply material assistance to those who seek high-tech medical services for the continuation or extension of life? (2) How should that public responsibility be discharged—through governmental or voluntary agencies? (3) How much of a priority should such pro-life procedures be accorded in the outlay of public finance, compared, for example, with expenses for such other needy categories as the unemployed, the blind, the disabled, etc.? (4) How should the potential beneficiaries be ranked—by what criteria? and (5) Who should be making these critical life-extending decisions?

While economic costs and scarcity pose the most immediate concerns in the arena of the "willing to live," other potential problems also should be noted. Many of these do not touch on the private/public sector relationships, but affect instead some of the traditional private law assumptions. How should the law treat the legal personality of one who has been implanted with another person's kidney or heart? And what if the transplanted body part is a sex organ or a whole head? When does a person cease to be one's self and becomes another? What about family relationships in such instances, and inheritance, and succession? Few of these questions have been even provisionally addressed this far. But the progress of biomedicine is not likely to slow down and a jurisprudential as well as a policy-making machinery will be necessary to sort out the great number of potential conflict areas created by man's inventiveness and the changes imposed by such inventions upon the natural world and its order.

The Willing to Procreate

The newest and most dramatic form of "wanted life" in contemporary society is that produced through artificial or surrogate parenting. Admittedly, in the course of history not all procreation occurred through the channels of the traditional family. Pregnancy by unwed mothers was prevalent in ancient times, and childbearing by concubines and slaves likewise served to produce a quasi-legitimate population growth.

But only in recent decades, however, have unwed women—and to a lesser extent men—set out in growing numbers to voluntarily undertake the task of single parenthood. What happens in these instances is a departure from traditional procreation, where two parents combine their decision-making, as well as resources, to provide for a new generation. The single parent is, indeed, accountable to no one in deciding to conceive, give birth and bring up a child. Parenting thus becomes a one-person proposition, not a familial balance.

The novelty of this new type of single person parenting, which differs from earlier known forms of single parenthood resulting from unforeseen and unplanned widowhood or divorce, is at times further enhanced by its initiation through artificial insemination. By foregoing carnal knowledge, the artificially-inseminated mother has a much wider choice of qualified fathers for the wanted child. The father can be selected from a wide range of options available at any semen bank. That father, however, might be totally unaware of the blessed conception and birth, and will remain without any input or responsibility for safeguarding the well-being of his own issue.

Recent years have seen a growing resort to even more innovative and high-tech procedures for parenting by those previously denied this privilege. Wed and unwed women who could not conceive, as well as married and unmarried men who could not impregnate, now find themselves participating in the child-bearing and child-raising process. Innovative technologies often permit both married and unmarried couples, not only to mutually produce a desired child, but also to resort to a third party as an intermediary for the final goal. Particularly noteworthy in this connection have been the functions of the surrogate mother who contracts to carry on a pregnancy for the benefit of another woman or couple. The "Baby M" controversy has demonstrated how profound the conflict is with regard, not only to surrogate mothering, but to other high-tech procedures as well. The judicial and legislative resolution of such cases is most troublesome.

These innovations in the interest of a wanted life have not only aroused the public's curiosities but have raised a growing number of moral and legal issues. In the first place, there has been little attention and even less discussion of society's policy towards deliberate single parenting. Should society sanction the practice? License it? Prohibit it?

In the next instance, one must seek to determine the responsibilities of all parties to the transaction—the deliberate mother and father, the contractual impregnator and the fetus carrier. Particularly in those situations where a third person enters into the relationship, such as a surrogate mother carrying a child intended for another couple, even more complex issues and conflicts are likely to arise. How valid legally and morally is a woman's contract consenting to be hired out as a surrogate mother? What are the relative rights of such a mother, carrying a fetus for nine months, against the woman who is to serve as a receiving parent? Should it matter that the fetus was parented by the husband of the receiving mother?

Above and beyond the rights of the involved parties, one must also address oneself to the interests of the community and the state. Not to be altogether overlooked, also, are the interests of the putative child—the life-to-be. Will society's needs be served by such unorthodox and complex means for child production? What prior scrutiny, if any, should be imposed upon potential parents, natural or surrogate? What assurances, if any, should be required of such parents that the potential child will indeed be the beneficiary of good parenting and the recipient of a good life? Given the economic as well as emotional costs to the parties entering into such unique contractual relationships and given the financial benefits derived by those fostering such contracts, isn't licensing or some state regulation necessary? Automobile drivers must conform to licensing, as do door-to-door solicitors in many jurisdictions. Many state legislatures have enacted laws which require regulation and licensing of surrogate organizations operating for profit. Moreover, several states prohibit outright such contractual relationships; the State of Michigan has gone so far as to make it a crime.

It would seem that an existing, constitutionally recognized "person" should not be free of public scrutiny and licensing when he or she sets out, with the aid of modern high-tech biomedicine, to produce another potential constitutional "person." It would appear that merely because these new "wanted life" procedures do not extinguish but rather create life should not exempt them from the quality of life considerations which have usually been directed to the unwanted life arena.

Conclusions: The Value of Human Life in a High-Tech World

It was observed in years gone by that the value of a human life cannot be measured by the market price of his component parts. Indeed, there is no accounting for the spiritual, intellectual, emotional and social value of any given human being. More recently, with the advance of the age of organ transplanting, the value of chemicals and organs contained in the human body has greatly escalated. With this escalation of humankind's physical components, what has occurred to a person's less tangible values?

Some fear that with growth of biomedical technology, our appreciation for the mystery of life and the uniqueness of creation are likely to diminish. Others point to the Nazi Holocaust and to subsequent human massacres as proof of the debasement of humanity. It has been suggested by still others that the leaps in technology and robotics make the human dispensable and might produce future trends for the debasement of human life. One must take notice of all these dire observations and predictions. But the responses and institutions required to counter all or any of the predicted adverse effects of the biomedical revolution cannot be readily shaped or articulated.

For the immediate future, one may be advised to seek more short-term solutions. Throughout history, the value of human life was manifested and protected through the institutions and practices of one's particular social environment: the family, tribe, village, or town. Many of these institutions, all through the world, have been losing their communal importance and vitality. As this

150

paper has sought to demonstrate, in many arenas of contemporary life, the role of the family has been drastically curtailed. There has been a decline in the role of the family regarding the decision to bear children, with regard to bringing them up and regarding the education of the young. Neither is the individual or family able to cope with the heavy burdens imposed by heroic medicine and the other tools for maintaining and extending life.

The whole arena of wanted life, in particular, must be reassessed to determine what new actors and institutions have been replacing or might replace those of old. What are the rights and responsibilities or these new actors—be they organ transplant banks, donors to artificial insemination centers or surrogate fathers and mothers? What is particularly noteworthy in the "wanted life" arena, with its commitment to the extension rather than extinction of life, is the growing realization that the pro-life forces have not granted this effort their whole-hearted support. In the pro-life camp there has been a tendency to overlook the new procedures' contribution to life and to dwell instead on their departure from, and disruption of, traditional institutions—such as marriage and the family. The traditional distinction between the pro-life and pro-quality of life persuasions thus appears to be based less on attitudes towards human life, as such, than on attitudes towards the *status quo* versus reform.

Hovering over all the individual actors and their considerations is the state, pursuing its own public policies and needs. It might be too early to foretell how all the diverse interests might be coordinated into a cohesive program which balances the interests of all or most of the concerned. It is clear, however, that the arena of "wanted life" is not totally free of conflict or of public policy disagreements. In the past half-century, the scholarly and judicial emphasis has been placed on "unwanted life," and to date that area continues to be rife with unresolved social, moral and jurisprudential questions rising from the arena of "wanted life," for "wanted life," much like "unwanted life," requires manipulations and changes in the natural order of living. What is eminently clear is that any departures from the traditional *status quo* cannot be attained without a considerable amount of social tension, compromise, and creative restructuring of our social institutions, as well as our individual lives.

EIGHT

HARD CHOICES

ETHICAL QUESTIONS RAISED BY THE BIRTH OF HANDICAPPED INFANTS

Helga Kuhse and Peter Singer

The Issue

We are now able to sustain the lives of many seriously ill or handicapped infants who, only a decade or two ago, would have died soon after birth because the means were not available to keep them alive. Not all seriously ill or handicapped infants will benefit from treatment, however. Some infants born very prematurely or with severe abnormalities cannot survive for long, despite the most aggressive efforts to keep them alive; others will survive with severe handicaps, either as part of their condition or as the result of efforts to sustain their lives.[1] With medicine's increased ability to delay or prevent death, an old question is raised with renewed urgency: Must every human life, regardless of its quality or kind, always be preserved, or are there times when an infant should be allowed, or helped, to die?

The following case will provide a background to these questions.

The Danville Siamese Twins

In May 1981, severely deformed Siamese twins were born in Danville, Illinois; the twins shared a lower body, intestinal tract, and had three legs between them—one normal leg each and a fused leg with too many toes. One of the twins had two holes in the heart. Both had trouble breathing and they had to be fed intravenously. The parents and their doctor decided that the twins should be allowed to die. However, against expectations, the twins did not die when medical treatment was withdrawn. When nourishment was withheld, an anonymous telephone caller alerted authorities and the parents and their doctor were subsequently charged with conspiracy to commit murder.[2]

The above case raises difficult ethical questions. Here are some of these questions:

- Does all human life have the same value? And should we always attempt to sustain life, irrespective of its quality?
- If life should not always be sustained, how severe must a handicap or abnormality be before life-sustaining treatment may be foregone?
- If the decision is made to withdraw or withhold treatment, should we merely allow the infant to die, or should we take positive steps to help him/her die?
- Who should make the decision? The parents? The doctors? The courts?
- Whose interests should be taken into account—only those of the infant or those of the family as well?

To discuss these questions adequately would require a book, not a single article.[3] Here we can do little more than show the problems, sketch our views and state the reasons why we hold them.

Does All Human Life Have the Same Value?

The "Sanctity-of-Life" View

People often say that human life has "sanctity." But what does "sanctity" mean and does all human life possess this sanctity equally? Not everyone who speaks of the "sanctity-of-life" subscribes to the same doctrine; rather, people hold a cluster of related ideas. Nevertheless, most supporters of the "sanctity-of-life" view agree in rejecting claims that one human life is more valuable than another. For Dr. Moshe Tendler, a professor of Talmudic law, all life is of *infinite* value:

> ...human life is of infinite value. This, in turn, means that a piece of infinity is also infinity, and a person who has but a few minutes to live is no less of value than a person who has but 60 years to live....a handicapped individual is a perfect specimen when viewed in an ethical context. The value is an absolute value. It is not relative to life expectancy, to state of health, or to usefulness to society.[4]

The Protestant theologian Paul Ramsey, professor of religion at Princeton University, takes a similar view:

> ...there is no reason for saying that six months in the life of a baby born with the invariably fatal Tay Sachs disease are a life-span of lesser worth to God than living 70 years before the onset of irreversible degeneration. A genuine humanist would say the same thing in other language. It is only a reductive naturalism or social utilitarianism that would regard those months of infant life as worthless because they lead to nothing on a time line of earthly achievement. All of our days and years are of equal worth whatever the consequence; death is no more a tragedy at one time than at another time.[5]

Not everybody believes that life has infinite value, that a day, hour, or even second of life is as valuable as a lifetime. Most of us would, we take it, be indifferent to our life being shortened by one second, but we are very far from indifferent to the thought that our life might be cut short by 10 or 20 years.

But there is another way of understanding the notion of the "sanctity-of-life." "Sanctity-of-life" is frequently understood to mean that all human life, irrespective of its quality or kind, is equally valuable. On this view, the life of a severely deformed Siamese twin or of a severely mentally-handicapped infant is no less valuable than that of a normal infant, or of any other patient.

The view that all human life has equal worth is deeply rooted in many people's prereflective thinking and is enshrined in the law. The central idea is well-expressed by Sanford Kadish when he describes the view of human life taken by Anglo-American law:

> All human lives must be regarded as having an equal claim to preservation, simply because life is an irreducible value. Therefore, the value of a particular life, over and above the value of life itself, may not be taken into account.[6]

This view of the equal value of all human lives was at the basis of the criminal charges instigated against the doctor and parents of the Danville Siamese twins. While the Illinois state attorney acknowledged that everyone may have acted from the best of motives when deciding that the infants should be allowed to die, he held:

> Motive has nothing to do with it. Quality of life has nothing to do with it. Under no circumstances do you take life because you disagree with the quality of it. These kids have lived and are human beings. They are entitled to life as long as nature gives it to them.[7]

And, when awarding custody of the twins to the Family Service Bureau, the judge agreed that he felt compassion for all involved, but also stated that it was not up to the Juvenile Court to make philosophical judgments:

> (The Court) must follow the Constitution of Illinois and of the United States, each of which contains a Bill of Rights. These Bills of Rights give every newborn Siamese twin with severe abnormalities an inalienable right to live.[8]

In this case, the court rejected quality-of-life considerations and upheld the equal value of all human life. As a consequence, two severely handicapped infants were kept alive against the wishes of the parents and irrespective of the infants' prospects to ever lead independent and minimally satisfying lives.

The view that all human life has equal worth may well be the simplest answer to the difficult issues raised about the treatment of infants born seriously ill or with major handicaps; but there are two questions that need to be asked about this simple answer: First, does anybody really believe that all human life has sanctity or equal worth and that the quality of the life in question does not count? Second, does this view have a sound, ethical basis? For the moment, we shall focus on the first question, leaving the theoretical issues for Section III.

156

Implicit quality-of-life judgments

The question of whether anybody really believes that all human life has equal worth was raised by the so-called "Baby-Doe Regulations," introduced by the Federal Government of the United States of America in 1982 to prevent discriminatory medical treatment of handicapped infants. The government was propelled into action by the death of "Baby Doe."

Baby Doe

Baby Doe was born on April 9, 1982, in Bloomington, Indiana, with Down's Syndrome and an esophageal atresia (the passage from the mouth to the stomach was not properly formed). Without surgery to repair the defect, such a baby will die. The prospects for successful surgery were fairly good but, even if surgery were performed, the baby's mental retardation would, of course, be unaffected. For this reason, the parents—supported by one of the doctors—decided against surgery. Baby Doe died on April 14, five days after his birth.[9]

Following Baby Doe's death, the Reagan Administration took steps to ensure that handicapped infants would not, in the future, be denied life-sustaining treatment.

In a "Notice to Health Care Providers" and the subsequent so-called "Baby-Doe Regulations," hospital administrators were reminded that it was unlawful under Section 504 of the Rehabilitation Act of 1973:

> for a recipient of Federal financial assistance to withhold from a handicapped infant nutritional sustenance or medical or surgical treatment required to correct a life-threatening condition if: (1) the withholding is based on the fact that the infant is handicapped; and (2) the handicap does not render treatment or nutritional sustenance contraindicated.[10]

In other words, the Reagan Administration suggested that no matter how severe an infant's handicap, the efforts made to preserve the baby's life must be no less than those made to preserve a non-handicapped infant's life in an otherwise similar condition. As Dr. C. Everett Koop, Surgeon General of the United States, put it when commenting on the government initiatives:

"This is a fight for a principle of this country—that every life is individually and uniquely sacred."[11]

But, American pediatricians were beginning to ask, did the guidelines require doctors to try to keep every infant alive—no matter what the prospects? To clarify this and other questions, the American Academy of Pediatrics took the Reagan Administration to court. When raising the question of the guideline's scope, the Academy referred to a number of conditions, including anencephaly (being born with most or all of the brain missing). Many of these babies die at birth or soon after, but some have lived for a week or two. With modern life-sustaining means, it would be possible to keep them alive for indefinite periods. But the absence, or virtual absence, of a brain means that even if such infants were to be kept alive, they would never be able to have conscious experiences, or respond in any way to other human beings.

Another condition mentioned by the Academy was one in which the infant lacks a substantial part of the digestive tract, for instance its intestine or bowels. The infant cannot be fed by mouth, for it will not obtain anything of nutritional value. It is not possible to correct the condition by surgery. Feeding such infants by means of an intravenous infusion directly into the bloodstream will keep them alive, but nutritional deficiencies are likely and the long-term prospects are poor.

At the Court hearing, the Department of Health and Human Services denied that doctors would be compelled to provide life-sustaining treatment in these extreme cases. The chief spokesperson for the Department's position was Dr. C. Everett Koop, himself an experienced pediatric surgeon and a supporter of the "Right-to-Life" movement. Referring to the case of a child having "essentially no intestine," Dr. Koop said:

> These regulations never intended that such a child should be put on hyper-alimentation (i.e., be artificially nourished) and carried for a year and a half. Incidentally, I was the first physician that ever did that, so I know whereof I speak. And we would consider customary care in that child the provision of a bed, of food by mouth, knowing that it was not going to be nutritious, but not just shutting off the care of that child....nor do we intend to say that this child should be carried on intravenous fluids for the rest of its life.

Dr. Koop made a similar remark about the other case mentioned by the Academy, that of an infant born with most or all of her brain missing:

> We would not attempt to interfere with anyone dealing with that child. We think it should be given loving attention and would expect it to expire in a short time.[12]

But Dr. Koop's view that these infants should not be kept alive is at odds with the belief that all human lives are of equal worth. For example, in the passage quoted above, Dr. Koop referred to the possibility of "carrying" an infant without an intestine for "a year-and-a-half;" yet Dr. Koop did not say that doctors should sustain an infant's life. But why not? Would he not think an 18-months' extension of life worthwhile for a normal child, or for a normal adult? If he would, the obvious explanation for his different view in the first case is that he does not regard the life of an artificially nourished infant as valuable as that of a normal infant or normal adult.

"Medical Decisions"

It is sometimes thought that the decision to refrain from employing life-sustaining procedures in the case of, say, infants born without intestines or brains is but a medical decision, which does not involve quality-of-life judgments. In its defense of the "Baby Doe Regulations," the Reagan Administration resorted to this type of argument.

When the Court found (on procedural grounds) in favor of the American Academy of Pediatrics, the Department of Health and Human Services issued a new "Proposed Rule" in July 1983. The new rule gave considerably more information on the circumstances in which it was to apply. In particular, it stated that "futile therapies, which merely temporarily prolong the process of dying" in an infant born with anencephaly or intra-cranial bleeding, need not be employed.

> Such medial decisions, by medical personnel and parents, concerning whether to treat, and if so what form the treatment should take, are outside the scope of Section 504.[13]

In other words, the Department suggested that in these cases, treatment is futile because it will only temporarily avert death; and what is "futile" is, according to the Department, a "medical decision."

But this will not do. Sophisticated modern techniques could indefinitely prolong the lives of children with anencephaly or intra-cranial bleeding. The judgment that someone whose life could indefinitely be prolonged by available medical means is "terminally ill" and, therefore, should not have his or her life prolonged is not a *medical* judgment; it is an ethical judgment about the desirability of prolonging that particular life.

Could the Department defend its view by saying that whether a patient is terminally ill is a medical judgment, based on the fact that the patient can survive only with the help of medical treatment? We think not. For if one were to take that view, then also a patient suffering from diabetes, would be "terminally ill" and doctors would not be required to provide "futile" therapy. The fact that no one in their right mind would regard insulin therapy as futile should make us realize that judgments about the futility of treatment are not purely medical judgments based on the prospects of extending the patient's life, but are rather judgments concerning the desirability of extending a life that is of a certain quality or kind.

Also the "Proposed Rule" has since been struck down by a Federal Court. The Department of Health and Human Services' appeal of this decision is at the time of writing still pending before the Supreme Court.

In the meanwhile, the Department has introduced a final rule under an amendment to the Child Abuse and Prevention Act. This rule, which is now in effect, recognizes a number of exceptions in the provision of life-sustaining treatment. It says, for example, that treatment is not required when "the infant is chronically and irreversibly comatose."[14] But this is, of course, again a quality-of-life judgment: a comatose infant's life need not be prolonged because comatose life is judged to be different and less valuable than conscious or self-conscious life.

Ordinary and Extraordinary Means

There is yet another way in which supporters of the view that all human lives are equally valuable make implicit quality-of-life judgments. This is the traditional Catholic distinction between ordinary and extraordinary means of treatment. Here it is claimed that there is no moral obligation to use "extraordinary means" of treatment; our obligations extend only to the provision of "ordinary means." Since it would require "extraordinary means" to keep alive an infant with virtually no brain or without an intestine, it is ethically acceptable to provide only ordinary care, and allow the infants to die.

The Catholic theologian Leonard Weber has discussed the ethical issues raised by the birth of seriously handicapped infants in his book *Who Shall Live?*[15] Weber explicitly rejects the view that decision-making ought to be based on quality-of-life considerations. A quality-of life approach, he says, offends against the equality of all human lives; the "extraordinary-means-approach," on the other hand, will offer some protection against an

> arbitrary decision being made on the basis of a judgment about the worth of a particular type of life. The decision will still be difficult and may still involve judgments about what constitutes successful treatment, but the focus on means is a constant reminder that we should not decide who should live or die on the basis of the worth of someone's life.[16]

What then is, according to Weber, extraordinary treatment? For handicapped infants, Weber holds, treatment is extraordinary or non-obligatory when it does not offer a reasonable hope of success, when it imposes an excessive burden in terms of, for example, repeated surgical interventions, or if such treatment leaves the child seriously handicapped:

> If, for example, the oxygen supply to the brain has been stopped and the opportunity to resuscitate such a person only comes when it is probable that extensive damage has already been done to the brain, it should be considered an extraordinary means to attempt to restore normal blood circulation, no matter how common the procedure.[17]

While Weber recognizes that others might want to say that nonresuscitation in this case involves a quality-of-life judgment, he nonetheless thinks it is the *treatment* which imposes an extraordinary burden. As he puts it, the child "would not have this burden if it were not for this treatment now."[18]

But the "burden" Weber speaks of is, of course, the infant's medical condition—the kind of life the infant will have after resuscitation. The future quality of the infant's life leads Weber to call the treatment "extraordinary" and hence, nonobligatory. But if that is so, then he is—regardless of the terminology used—making a quality-of-life judgment.

Quality-of-life criteria are also implicit in the now classical definition, by the Jesuit theologian Gerald Kelly, of "extraordinary treatment" as:

> all medicines, treatments and operations, which cannot be obtained without excessive expense, pain or inconvenience, or which, if used, would not offer a reasonable hope of benefit.[19]

Take the terms "excessive" or "benefit." How do we determine whether a life-sustaining treatment is excessively expensive or burdensome, or whether it will benefit a particular patient? Initially, we might want to say that a treatment benefits a patient if it sustains her life. But is a longer life always of benefit to a patient? We think not—and neither do those who rely on the distinction between ordinary and extraordinary means. Whether a treatment is of benefit depends on the patient's medical condition and on whether it can provide the patient with an acceptable quality of life. Even the Catholic Church acknowledges this when, in the Vatican's *Declaration on Euthanasia*, it is stated that it might be better to speak not of "extraordinary" but of "disproportionate means" of treatment.[20] But when is a treatment disproportionately expensive or burdensome—or, in the language of Gerald Kelly—"excessively" so? Quite clearly, the answer to this question will vary in accordance with the patient's medical condition, with the quality and quantity of life available to the patient with or after treatment. An unpleasant operation, for example, might be disproportionately burdensome for a terminally-ill patient because it will extend an already burdensome life by only a short period. On the other hand, if a patient were by the same operation to gain another 20 or 30 years of normal life, then the operation would not be disproportionately burdensome.

The upshot is that the distinction between ordinary and extraordinary means (or between proportionate and disproportionate means) has little to do with "means"—considered simply as means—but much with the prospects of particular patients, including the patient's prospective quality of life.

We conclude that even those who claim that all human life is of equal worth do not, in practice, take this rhetoric seriously.

Can the claim be defended that all human life is of equal worth? We do not think so. In the following, we state our reasons for that view.

Why We Should Reject the Sanctity-of-Life View

What's special about human life?

We have already noted that even those who speak of the "sanctity-of-life" do not take their rhetoric seriously. In various ways, quality-of-life considerations enter into their life and death decisions. We should, however, also notice something else. Those who speak of the "sanctity-of-life" do not really mean to say that *all* life is sacred or has the same value. It is *human* life which they see as sacred; they are not generally saying that the life of a sheep, chicken, earthworm or lettuce has the same value as the life of a human being. While this may seem quite obvious, we should keep this fact in mind because it will remind us that even those who want to rank all *human* life equally are making different judgments about the value of different lives. The fact that they are making such judgments entitles us to ask what the distinctions are based on; or, to put the question differently, what *is* it that gives value to human life, but not—or not to the same degree—to the lives of other living things?

Two answers are possible. The first answer is that human life has sanctity simply because it is *human* life, that is, because it is the life of a member of the species *homo sapiens.* The second answer is that human life has special value because humans are rational, autonomous, purposeful, moral beings, with hopes, ambitions, life-purposes, ideals, and so on. Any of these qualities, or a combination of them, could serve as the basis for a moral distinction between human beings and lettuces or chickens. That such distinguishing qualities are needed is clear: for if the value of life were based on mere "life," rather than on one or more of the above characteristics, every life—including the earthworm's or the lettuce's—would be equally valuable.

It is not difficult to see that the second answer does point to a morally relevant difference between some lives and others. For example, it is quite plausible to hold that the life of a self-aware, rational, purposeful being that sees itself as existing over time is more valuable than the life of an entity or being who lacks these characteristics. But here we must note the following: if one takes this approach, then one is not saying that human *life* has sanctity, but rather that rationality, the capacity to be moral or purposeful, the capacity for the holding of ideals, and so on, has "sanctity." Of course, one may still hold that human life has sanctity or special value, but only insofar as bodily life is a precondition for rationality, purposiveness, or whatever else one takes the valuable characteristic to be. One would *not*, on this view, be able to argue that the lives of all members of the human species have special value—for example, the lives of the irreversibly comatose, or the lives of those who are not and never will be rational and purposive beings.

In the context of a discussion concerning the treatment of handicapped infants, it is also important to note that no newly-born infant—whether handicapped or not—is a rational, pur-posive or moral being. Most infants do possess the potential to develop these characteristics. But this raises the separate question of whether we should treat a being on the basis of its actual characteristics, or its potential. Leaving this issue aside for the moment, we also must note that unfortunately some newborn infants do not even possess the potential to develop these char-acteristics. Anencephalic infants and some severely brain dam-aged or retarded infants fall into this category.

The second approach, then, does not give us a reason for preserving the lives of all human infants and cannot serve as the basis for the view that *all* human lives, irrespective of their quality or kind, are equally valuable.

The first answer does cover all human infants—by definition. But can the fact that a being belongs to the species *homo sapiens,* rather than to another species, tell us anything about the value of that being's life? In our view it cannot. The difference to which it points is simply a difference in species. Nothing is said as to why species should matter. While it may initially seem obvious that human life is more valuable than nonhuman life, it is also "obvious" to the racist or sexist that a person's race or sex should determine how that person ought to be treated. But just as race or sex are not morally relevant in themselves, neither is species. If we say that the lives of beings of our own species are valuable, but the lives of beings of other species are not, *merely because these beings do not belong to our species,* then on what basis can we criticize the racist who says that beings of his or her race have special value, but beings of other races do not? We believe that neither race nor species are morally relevant in themselves. What matters are a being's capacities—the kind of life a being has.

This conclusion should, in our view, also be applied to severely handicapped infants. We should not argue that they must have their lives sustained because they are human. We must ask what kind of beings they are and what kind of life they have.

It is not life which has value, but only life of a certain quality.

Consistently applied, the "sanctity-of-life" view does not allow any quality-of-life judgments. In other words, on this view life would have to be prolonged even if the patient would not benefit from such efforts. On example would be the extension of an infant's life in a situation where that infant—either because it is born without a brain or has suffered severe brain damage after birth—will never be able to have conscious experiences. While such an infant will not experience pain or suffering, neither will it experience pleasure or joy—or any of the things that make life valuable. Its life would be like a dreamless sleep. Would it be of value to the infant to have its life prolonged? We think not—for the infant cannot be benefitted by anything we do.

In this case, life would be of *no* value to the infant. Are there also situations where life can be a disvalue? This question is raised by the following case which is in some ways similar to that of Baby Doe.

Brian West

Brian West was born in October 1980 to Susan and John West. Brian was born with Down's Syndrome and a severe form of esophageal atresia, that is, there was no connection between the back of his mouth and his stomach. Doctors recommended surgery to construct a new esophagus. Brian's parents refused consent for the operation, and the court took custody of Brian and ordered sufficient medical treatment to keep him alive. During the next 26 months, Brian's treatment involved, at different times, the attachment of a permanent abdominal feeding tube, the insertion of a breathing tube in his mouth, and the attachment of an intravenous needle to his neck. When, in November 1982, the reconstructive surgery was finally performed, Brian weighed only 15 lbs. He responded to the surgery with respiratory shock, a massive blood infection, and temporary kidney failure. John West gave the following account:

> Whenever we visited him during this time, he was screaming in pain. He was tied spread-eagle in his hospital crib for six weeks to keep him from pulling at his surgical wounds. I don't think he ever recovered from this. When the wounds healed, he never showed the same level of alertness or interest in toys as he did before the surgery. He had recurring episodes of pain as gastric juices backed up into his esophagus (it lacked the valve which is normally present to prevent this). He continued to have numerous bouts with pneumonia.[21]

> In November 1982, Brian went into hospital because of breathing problems. He became unconscious and was placed on a respirator. When taken off the respirator, Brian was found to have suffered brain damage and to be blind. He spent five weeks in intensive care.

> Whenever he was awake, he was agitated and writhing in his bed...The doctors told us they had no idea whether he was in pain or not, but one look at him made your whole body cringe...On December 21, 1982, thank God, he died. We loved Brian and we always wanted the best for him.[22]

If all human life were of infinite or equal value, there would be no point in considering whether everything possible should always be done to keep an infant alive. But the above case raises just this issue.

Considering Brian's life from his point of view—disregarding entirely what his parents went through, and the cost of his medical care—it would have been better if he had died shortly after birth. Extended periods of his life were wrought with pain and suffering, so whatever better moments he may have had in his short existence cannot have compensated for them. Those who obtained the court order to save Brian's life did no good; on the contrary, they did him great harm.

Looking back over Brian's life now that it is over, this judgment seems undeniable; but could one argue that at the time when the court order was granted, it was in Brian's interests to have the surgery carried out? After all, it was not then apparent how bad the outcome would be. It *might* have succeeded. Was the risk worthwhile?

In taking any risk, we weigh the possible benefits against the possible costs, and try to assess the probability of each. Here, the fact that we are dealing with *infants*, rather than with older children or adults, is relevant.

Infants and Persons

Unlike an older child or adult, an infant cannot choose whether or not to undergo prolonged, invasive and sometimes painful life-sustaining treatment—whether she would want to undergo the pain and suffering to gain a few more months of life, a year, or a life-time. Does this mean that we must always attempt to sustain the infant's life, or should we allow infants like Brian West, Baby Doe and the Siamese twins to die?

This question cannot be answered, we believe, until we have reflected on the issue of what it is that distinguishes the lives of newborn infants from the lives of older children and adults.

Adults and children—but not infants—are self-aware and purposeful beings with a sense of the past and the future: they can see their lives as a continuing process; they can identify with what has happened to them in the past, and they have hopes and plans for the future. For this reason we can say that, in normal circumstances, continued life is what they want, and is in their interests. Newborn infants are not capable of seeing their lives in this way. They can have no desire to continue to live, because they have no concept of their own future life. There are no links, either of memory or of anticipation, between the separate moments of their existence. This means that, strictly speaking, we cannot even say that continued life is in their interests; for while it may be true that a newborn infant will, if all goes well, grow into a happy child and lead a worthwhile life, that later life is not linked, at the mental level, with the life of the infant. The infant and the child or adult are physically the same organism, but the child is a *person*, in the full sense of the term, and a newborn infant is not.

We shall use the term "person" to refer to those who understand that they exist over time with a past and a possible future. The lives of persons can be seen as journeys on which they have embarked. Although we know that the final destination must be death, there are goals along the way which we are hoping to achieve before the trip is over. Extending a person's life through medical technology will normally extend the journey and increases the possibilities of reaching some of these goals. The value of life-saving procedures is especially apparent in a case where accident or illness threatens to cut off the journey when it has still some way to go, and so thwarts the fulfillment of hopes and desires which might otherwise have been realized.

It might be objected that our journey begins with birth, or even conception; that death *in utero* or shortly after birth is the worst possible fate, for it ensures that none of the goals which might have been achieved will ever be reached. But this is a mistake. The journey is not underway in any purposeful sense, for the fetus or the newborn infant is not aware of itself as a being with a past and a future. The fetus or infant has no goals, no hopes, no expectations. This means that the journey we have talked about gets under way only some time after birth when there is a being capable of seeing itself as a traveler, and capable of wanting to reach some goal, however simple that goal might be. If this is correct, then it also must be correct that the loss of life for a newly-born infant is, other things being equal, much less significant than the loss of life for an older child or adult.

This conclusion has far-reaching consequences for the difficult questions we raised at the beginning; but before we come to these, we shall consider an objection to what we have just said, for the objection helps to clarify our position. This objection relates to the infant's potential.

The argument from potential and the infant's best interests

We have claimed that the death of a fetus or infant does not have the same moral significance as the death of an older child or adult because there are no hopes which will go unrealized, and no goals which will not be reached. But, someone might object, a fetus or infant—and this includes many handicapped infants—have the potential to have, and realize many of the goals that we have been speaking about. It is the loss of that potential—the fact that, to invoke our metaphor, the whole journey will never be made—which constitutes the tragedy in the death of a fetus or infant. Compared with such a loss, it scarcely matters whether the hopes and desires ever have been consciously felt.

This argument from potential is sometimes invoked to justify aggressive treatment of seriously ill or handicapped infants. If the treatment succeeds, so the argument goes, the future child or adult will be grateful that her life was saved and that many of her plans and goals can now be realized. Hence, a supporter of this view might say, it was in the infant's interest to undergo the treatment.

Based on this view, many people believe that the guiding principle should be "the best interests of the infant." Life-sustaining treatment should be given to an infant if her future life, with or after treatment, would contain more benefits than burdens. This view is, for example, taken by the United States President's Commission for the Study of Ethical Problems in Medicine and Biomedical and Behavioral Research in its report *Deciding to Forego Life-Sustaining Treatment*.[23] While this view has an obvious appeal, there are a number of reasons as to why we think we should not accept it. The most important reasons have to do with the special status of infants.

Let us begin by asking: "What *are* the interests of an infant?" Obviously, a newborn infant can feel pain, be cold and hungry; it can, therefore, be said to have an interest in not experiencing pain, to be warm and well-fed. But those who suggest that decision-making should be based on the "best interests of the infant" are looking much further ahead than this. They are thinking of the whole future of the infant, and whether the future life will, in its totality, contain more benefits than harms for the child or adult into which the child will develop.

There is, however, a problem in seeing life five years hence, no matter how good a life it may be, as in the interests of *this* infant lying here in front of us. Suppose that if we continue treatment there is a good chance that this infant will, in five years, be a normal child playing in the sandpit with her friends. Suppose that we do continue treatment, everything works out as we had hoped, and the child is brought back to see us, clearly enjoying life as much as any five-year-old. Can we then think back to the day we stood before the newborn infant, wondering whether to operate, and say to ourselves, "In that case, at least, treatment was in the best interests of the infant?" Before we say this, we ought to ask, "In what sense is the child I see before me now *the same person* as the infant who was then in the neo-natal intensive care unit?"

There is, of course, a physical continuity between the child and the infant. The latter developed into the former. Because of this, they may be said to be the same physical organism, despite the great changes that have taken place. But there is no mental continuity. The child cannot look back and recall the time she was an infant in the neo-natal intensive care unit. Nor could the infant look forward to the time when she would be an older child.

This is not a simple matter of a limit to the length of recall of the child, or the range of anticipation of the infant. It is not as if the child can now remember being a two-year-old, and the two-year-old could remember her first birthday, and the child who had just turned one could remember the first weeks of her life. If there were this kind of overlapping continuity, it would be possible to say that the infant and the five-year-old are the same person, just as a rope made up of overlapping strands would still be one rope, even though no single strand reached from one end to the other. But we have *no* conscious links with our infancy, because as an infant we were not beings with the kind of awareness necessary for spanning time.[24]

This makes it very dubious to claim that the happy child shows that a decision to continue treatment was in "the best interests of the infant." It may show that the decision was justified because. among other things, it made possible the enjoyable and worthwhile life now being lived by the child; but this is a different matter. The infant has no interest in becoming that child; its interests are much more limited than that: not to suffer, to be warm and comfortable, and so on. If the infant has good prospects of intact survival, but the form of treatment required will cause prolonged pain and discomfort, we may have to recognize that we are doing it, not in accordance with, but *despite* "the best interests of the infant."

This issue is raised starkly in the context of infants born prematurely, at the margin of viability. In many cases, doctors will not give anesthetics for invasive treatments, including major surgery, because this would put an additional strain on the infant's immature system, thereby threatening the infant's chances of survival. But this practice—one doctor calls it a "barbarism"[25] — is surely not in the infant's best interests. If this is correct, this means that in some extreme cases the suffering of the infant—unavoidable if it is to be kept alive—may in itself be sufficient reason to forego the treatment. The situation of Brian West may have been one such case.

Moreover, if the argument is that treatment, including very painful treatment, can be justified because it is likely to result in the existence of a person who, five or 20 years from now, will be glad to be alive, then we must also consider the issues from yet another perspective: that of abortion and even nonconception, both of them widely accepted. In other words, if the argument is that it would be *wrong* to let an infant die because this would result in there not being—in five or 20 years' time—a person leading a worthwhile life, then the same argument would lead to the condemnation of not only abortion but also nonconception. In both cases, there is the loss of a possible life—a journey which will never be made, a life which will never be lived.

Here, we should note that our concern is not to deny that, other things being equal, it is a good thing to bring additional human beings into existence—at least if they can be expected to have lives above a certain minimal quality; but this conclusion gives us no reason to see the death of a fetus or newborn infant—from the future person's perspective—as more tragic than anything else which prevents the existence of such a person.

This answers the objection. What we must now do is ask, "Whose interests should be taken into account when we make life and death decisions for a seriously ill or handicapped infant?"

In Whose Interests?

In the last section, we sketched the philosophical difficulties that lurk behind the idea that decision-making should be based on "the best interests of the infant." These difficulties are one reason as to why we think this approach is misguided. There is, however, also another more straightforward reason: many other factors should, in our view, be taken into account—including the interests of the parents, and of any children they may already have. It is, for example, often pointed out that the survival of a handicapped child is also the creation of a handicapped family. While the judgment may be too severe in some cases, in others it is the simple truth.[26]

There is no reason to assume that the interests of the child or person who the handicapped infant might become should automatically outweigh all these other interests. The birth of a severely handicapped infant can dramatically change the lives of the parents and siblings. To disregard their interests altogether is incompatible with the principle of equal consideration of the interests of all those affected by our decision—and such a principle is fundamental to ethics.

If we speak about consideration of interests, there is also one other interest which we have not, so far, raised: the "interests" of the next child in the queue.

One of the more firmly established findings about families with a disabled child is that they are less likely than other families to have further children.[27] Shouldn't we take the interests of those children into account—the interests of the children who will not exist if the handicapped infant survives?

Peggy Stinson is an American woman who has published a book called *The Long Dying of Baby Andrew*. The book is based on a journal she kept during the period when doctors were, against her wishes, trying to save Andrew's life—despite the fact that he was highly unlikely to survive without severe brain damage. Peggy Stinson's journal shows that, like most mothers in her situation, she was concerned about what Andrew's long-term survival in a damaged state might do to her plans to have another child. On February 17, when Andrew was two months old, she wrote:

> I keep thinking about the other baby—the one that won't be born. The IICU [Infant Intensive Care Unit] is choosing between lives. It may already be too late for the next baby. If Andrew's life is strung out much longer, will we have the money, the emotional resources, the nerve to try again?[28]

The journal entry for April 30, 1977 is particularly interesting because it poses the philosophical question that is at the hub of this issue:

> Thirty-fifth birthday coming next week; haven't got forever to try for another child. If we wait much longer, until our insurance runs out or we're billed for Andrew's custodial care, we'll know we can't afford another child. Or we won't have the nerve to try again. We want another child. I'm not going to let Pediatric Hospital [where Andrew was kept alive against his parents' wishes] destroy our chance to have one. At this rate we'll have neither Andrew nor the next child, who, because of Andrew's extended course, will have lost the chance to exist at all.

> Jeff [a junior doctor at the hospital more sympathetic to the Stinsons' view than the other senior medical staff] once said our "next child" was theoretical, abstract—its interests couldn't be considered. Strictly speaking that may be so, but the next baby seems real enough to me. To Bob, too. Decision this week to change that abstraction into a real person before it's too late.[29]

Is the "next child" an abstraction whose interests cannot be considered before it is born, or even conceived?

The argument that we should take the "next child" into account has been well put by R.M. Hare, in a discussion of abortion of a fetus known to have a handicap.[30] Hare points out that in such discussions one interest is frequently overlooked: the interest of "the next child in their queue." Suppose, he says, that a couple have planned to have two children. The second child is discovered, during pregnancy, to have a serious handicap. If the fetus lives, the couple will not have any more children. If the fetus is aborted, the couple will seek to have a second child. There is a high probability that this second child will be normal. In this situation, Hare argues, we should consider not only the interests of the child now in the womb, but also the interests of the possible child who is likely to live if, and only if, this child does not live.

This account can be applied to the situation of the severely handicapped newborn infant. Here, too, couples are often likely to have a further child only if the newborn infant does not live.[31] Should we exclude this fact from our deliberations of whether to treat a handicapped infant? We think we should not—at least not if we believe that treatment is justified in terms of the interests of the future child or person. There is, of course, another reason as well: the pain and suffering that will sometimes have to be inflicted if we want to ensure the survival of a seriously ill or handicapped infant.

Who Should Decide?

There is now general agreement that adult, competent patients—not the doctor—should decide whether they want to undergo certain treatment, including life-sustaining treatment. But who should make the decision whether or not a severely handicapped infant lives? There have been proposals, especially in the United States, for ethics committees—or even courts—to decide difficult cases.

But committees or courts are hardly well-suited to the type of urgent decision-making which can be required, at any hour of the day or night, in a neo-natal intensive care unit. Moreover, there is a fundamental objection to this way of making decisions put by Robert and Peggy Stinson in their book about the treatment of Baby Andrew:

> We believe there is a moral and ethical problem of the most fundamental sort involved in a system which allows complicated decisions of this nature to be made unilaterally by people who do not have to live with the consequences of their decisions.[32]

We agree. It cannot be right for others to override the desire of parents that their extremely handicapped baby should not live, and then to return that infant to the unwilling parents, with all the consequences that bringing up such a child may have for them and their other children. It would be different if there were other couples willing to adopt the child, or if the community were prepared to pay for the kind of institutional care that would be needed for the child to have a good life; unfortunately, very few couples are willing to adopt severely handicapped children, and institutional care is almost everywhere far below the standard required. In virtually every case, the infant's best, and usually only, chance of a decent life is with the parents. In these circumstances, the parents' views about treatment should be decisive.

We recognize that the birth of a handicapped infant can be a great shock to the parents, and it will sometimes be difficult for them to make such important decisions immediately after birth. However, in a well-known article, two pediatricians have reported their experience that parents, regardless of background, can make informed, understanding decisions if they are carefully and sympathetically told the facts in words they can understand.[33] We see no reason to doubt this. We also think that the situation could be ameliorated if, as another pediatrician William Silverman, has suggested, obstetricians were to discuss with expectant parents the possibility of the baby being born handicapped, seriously ill or extremely prematurely, and the need to make decisions about treatment in such circumstances.[34] Such discussions would arouse less anxiety if they were perfectly routine, taking place perhaps at prenatal classes.

Conclusion

We have argued that parents should, other things being equal, decide whether their severely handicapped infant lives or dies. One issue we have not raised is *how* the infant should die.

Many people draw a moral distinction between doing something that results in death, or between killing and letting die. Thus, it is often thought that letting die is sometimes permissible, but killing never. Based on this distinction, doctors will frequently decide not to act to preserve the life of handicapped infants—such as the Danville Twins and Baby Doe—but not take active steps to end the infants' lives.

We deny that there is a moral distinction between killing and letting die. If all other factors, such as motivation and outcome, are the same, killing and letting die are morally equivalent. Does this mean it does not matter whether an infant is killed or allowed to die? We do not think so. To the extent that letting die can often be a drawn out and distressing process for all concerned—including, of course, the infant—we think that there are circumstances where severely ill or handicapped infants should not only be allowed to die, but should be helped to die.

ACKNOWLEDGEMENTS

Parts of this article are drawn from a book: *Should the Baby Live?*, Oxford University Press, 1985; selections of the article are also drawn from an article "Ethical Issues Raised by the Birth of Extremely Premature Infants," in [eds.] V. Yu and C. Wood: *Prematurity*, published by Churchill Livingstone in 1987.

NOTES

1. See, for example, Helga Kuhse and Caroline de Garis (eds.), *Proceedings of the Conference: The Tiniest Newborns, Survival—What Price?* (Melbourne: Centre for Human Bioethics, Monash University, 1984).
2. News Item, *Independent Journal,* June 13, 1981; News Item, *The Age* [Melbourne], June 8, 1981; John A. Robertson, "Dilemma in Danville," *The Hastings Center Report,* vol. 11, 1981, 5–8.
3. See Helga Kuhse and Peter Singer, *Should the Baby Live? The Problem of Handicapped Infants,* (Oxford, New York, Melbourne: Oxford University Press, 1985 and 1986).
4. Moshe Tendler, as cited by Edward Keyserlingk, *Sanctity of Life or Quality of Life, in the Context of Ethics, Medicine, and Law: A Study Written for the Law Reform Commission of Canada* (Ottawa: Law Reform Commission, 1979), 31.
5. Paul Ramsey, *Ethics at the Edges of Life* (New Haven and London: Yale University Press, 1978), 191.
6. Sanford H. Kadish, "Respect for Life and Regard for Rights in the Criminal Law," in S.F. Barker (ed.), *Respect for Life in Medicine, Philosophy, and the Law,* (Baltimore and London: The Johns Hopkins University Press, 1977), 72.
7. Robertson, "Dilemma in Danville," *op. cit.*
8. *Ibid.*
9. For the medical history of Baby Doe, see the letter to the editor by John E. Pless, M.D., of Bloomington Hospital, *New England Journal of Medicine,* vol. 309, September 15, 1983, 664.
10. See Helga Kuhse and Peter Singer, *Should the Baby Live?, op. cit.,* 20–30.
11. C. Everett Koop, as cited by James Rachels, *The End of Life* (Oxford, New York, Melbourne: Oxford University Press, 1986), 64.

12. The statements by Dr. C. Everett Koop can be found in the transcript of the proceedings before the United States District Court for the District of Columbia, *American Academy of Pediatrics, et. al. v. Margaret Heckler, Secretary, Department of Health and Human Services*, Washington, D.C., Civil Action no. 83-0774 [March 21, 1983], 44–45.

13. Helga Kuhse and Peter Singer, *Should the Baby Live?, op. cit.*, 27ff.

14. See John C. Moskop and Rita L. Saldanha, "The Baby Doe Rule: Still a Threat," *Hastings Center Report*, vol. 16, April 1986, 8–14.

15. Leonard Weber, *Who Shall Live?* (New York, Ramsey, Toronto: Paulist Press, 1976).

16. *Ibid.*, 85.

17. *Ibid.*, 92–93.

18. *Ibid.*, 93.

19. Gerald Kelly, S.J., *Medico-Moral Problems* (St. Louis: The Catholic Hospital Association), 129.

20. Sacred Congregation for the Doctrine of the Faith, *Declaration on Euthanasia*, Vatican City, 1980, 10–11.

21. Helga Kuhse and Peter Singer, *Should the Baby Live?, op. cit*, 142.

22. *Ibid.*

23. President's Commission for the Study of Ethical Problems in Medicine and Biomedical and Behavioral Research, *Deciding to Forego Life-Sustaining Treatment, Ethical, Medical, and Legal Issues in Treatment Decisions* (Washington: US Government Printing Office, 1983), chapter 6.

24. See Michael Tooley, *Abortion and Infanticide* (Oxford: Oxford University Press, 1983), chapter 5.

25. John W. Scanlon, M.D., "Barbarism," *Pre-natal Press*, vol. 9, no. 7, 1985.

26. See, e.g., Stephen Kew, *Handicap and Family Crisis* (London: Pittman, 1975).

27. *Ibid.*, 52.

28. Robert and Peggy Stinson, *The Long Dying of Baby Andrew* (Boston and Toronto: An Atlantic Monthly Press Book, Little, Brown and Company, 1983), 153.

29. *Ibid.*, 266–267.

30. R.M. Hare, "Survival of the Weakest" in S. Gorovitz, et. al., *Moral Problems in Medicine* (Englewood Cliffs: Prentice Hall, 1976), 369–375.

31. Stephen Kew, *Handicap and Family Crisis, op. cit.*

32. Peggy and Robert Stinson, "On the Death of a Baby," *Atlantic Monthly*, July 1979, as cited by Helen Harrison with Ann Kositsky, R.N.: *The Premature Baby Book* (New York: St. Martin's Press, 1983), 103.

33. R. Duff and A.G.M. Campbell, "Moral and Ethical Dilemmas in the Special-Care Nursery," *New England Journal of Medicine*, vol. 2898, October 23, 1973, 885–894.

34. Michael O'Donnell, "One Man's Burden," *British Medical Journal*, vol. 286, April 16, 1983, 1291.

NINE

The APPROPRIATE MEDICAL CARE Of the TERMINALLY ILL

Jan Kryspin and Heather Phillips

The human condition, of its very nature, is a terminal condition. Thus it was contemplated in poignant imagery by an unknown companion of the 7th century Anglo-Saxon king, Edwin.

> This is how the present life of man on earth, King, appears to me in comparison with that time which is unknown to us. You are sitting feasting with your ealdormen and thegns in wintertime; the fire is burning on the hearth in the middle of the hall and all inside is warm, while outside the wintry storms of rain and snow are raging; and a sparrow flies swiftly through the hall. It enters in at one door and quickly flies out through the other. For the few moments it is inside, the storm and wintry tempest cannot touch it, but after the briefest moment of calm, it flits from your sight, out of the wintry storm and into it again. So this life of man appears but a moment.[1]

In the 20th century such a view, though real enough to those who stand at death's door (the elderly and the terminally ill), is no longer publicly acceptable.

Indeed, it is well-known that in 20th-century Western society, death has replaced sex as the great taboo. While more than a million human beings die on this planet each week, mostly from age and terminal illness of one sort or another, and while in the private lives of ordinary people where death occurs, there are countless painful explosions of grief and deep human response, in public we do not die.[2] No longer are we supported by the social customs of millennia, which placed death in perspective as part of the collective cycle of human life.[3] Because the ethos of our culture is so deeply pervaded by materialism, by the priority of material well-being, we experience a collective need to preserve the appearance of happiness. Real death, real grief, the terminal condition of all of us, is no longer acknowledged in the collective public awareness.

Historically speaking, this denial of our terminal condition is a very recent phenomenon. In the world of our ancestors, life was short. The average age of the population of England in the early 19th century was less than 30 (comparable to that of modern day Sri Lanka). A mere 7 percent of men and women lived beyond the age of 60, as compared with some 20 percent in present-day England.[4] That world, now lost to us, was a world full of children; crowds of little children, playing in the village streets and farmyards, crowding around the cottage fires. In Stuart England, for example, 45 percent of all the people alive were children.[5] And (paradoxically to us) that world of the young was a world where death was ever present. People were used to bereavement. They had to be because it happened all the time. What we consider to be "natural death," that is, death as a gradual fading away in old age, was the exception rather than the rule. Death by accident, drowning, pleurisy or the plague, pointed out the philosopher Montaigne in 1580, was far more "natural" because it was general, common and universal.[6]

Modern medicine succeeded in all but abolishing death. For most people, premature death no longer lies just around the corner. Life expectancy has increased. The death of infants, children and young adults is now so unlikely as to be virtually unthinkable. Those who die are mostly old (over 80 percent of us). And the nature of terminal illness has changed. Bubonic plague, smallpox, tuberculosis and other communicable diseases have given way to chronic degenerative diseases—cardiovascular disorders, cancer, arthritis and respiratory diseases (including bronchitis and emphysema). We all die sooner or later. Most of us nowadays expect that it will be later. Most live into old age in a state of chronic disease, our natural forces slowly running down, with an indeterminate amount of time ahead of us—the senescent ill. But for some, who succumb to severe life-threatening illness, the time ahead is more or less limited and determined—the terminally ill. (The two categories are, of course, by no means altogether separate.) The circumstances which have brought about the prolongation of life and the existence of the senescent ill as a significant part of the population in 20th-century Western society—advances in medical science and technology—have brought about also a subtle transformation in our perception of our allotted time, and hence, in our idea of death. Death, it is commonly held, need not occur in the foreseeable future. It is a postponable event. Thus, the reality of our basic human condition—our terminal condition—is obscured. This failure to simply and appropriately acknowledge our terminal condition is the source of our deepest problem in caring for the terminally ill.

The classic statement of the aim and scope of medicine: "to cure rarely, to relieve sometimes, to comfort always," reflects the balance and sanity of a more tranquil age than our own, an age in which men and women lived in full awareness of their terminal condition. Health, in our culture, tends to be perceived as "a struggle against death by escalating application of industrial power."[7] And thus, the modern hospital with its advanced technology and specialist expertise is geared towards investigation, diagnosis, cure and prolonging of life. In such a cure-oriented, death-defying environment the dying patient is, inevitably, perceived as a failure of the healthcare system. The result, for such a patient, is isolation and intensified suffering. While every effort is made to obstruct the sparrow's passage, there is certainly no time to contemplate the mystery of its existence.

Totally out of step with the common attitude down the ages, Western medicine's practical denial of the human condition has resulted, in the last 10 years, in a reactionary phenomenon of remarkable vigor and vitality—the hospice movement, oriented toward comfort rather than cure, with its humane goal of symptom control aimed at providing optimum quality of life for the dying. In North America alone, hospices now number in the hundreds, and the literature is vast.[8] "Hospice" was originally a medieval name for a stopping place on the way, where pilgrims and travelers could receive comfort and hospitality. And the hospice ideal is, clearly, an attempt to recover the traditional, age-old awareness of death—death as part of life itself, a mystery to be contemplated rather than a problem to be attacked by medical intervention. It may be, however, that there is still more of value in the care of the terminally ill to be learned from the past.

Ethical Principles

Currently, in the English-speaking world, there would appear to be four "cardinal principles" in use in medical ethics: Patient autonomy, Beneficence, Non-maleficence and Justice.[9] How such principles are applied to the care of the terminally ill has been recently demonstrated by Dr. Edmund Pellegrino, Director of the Kennedy Institute of Ethics in Washington, at the Sixth World Congress on Care of the Terminally Ill (Montreal, September–October 1986). In a compelling paper, Dr. Pellegrino outlined a comprehensive scheme for deciding what is in the best interests of the terminally ill patient. The guiding principle of his scheme was Beneficence: how do we help and heal this particular patient, recognizing that helping and healing do not stop even though we have made a diagnosis of terminal illness and a hopeless future? The distinction between what is legal and what is ethical (a distinction nowadays often blurred) always must be kept in mind. An ethical, morally defensible treatment of the terminally ill patient must proceed with due deference to the personhood and humanity of the patient and of all involved in the decision making process. (In a pluralistic society, neither the patient nor any member of the healthcare team may impose his or her values on one another.) Thus, Pellegrino's starting point was the concept of patient autonomy—the competent patient can and should decide for himself how his treatment should proceed. In the U.S., since the Quinlan case (1976), the courts have upheld the principle of autonomy—the legal and moral right to decide how one will live one's life and/or end it. For the incompetent patient, Pellegrino outlined a framework of alternatives for substitute judgment: by anticipatory declaration, living will, durable power of attorney, or other verifiable statement by the patient of what he would have wanted had he been able to speak for himself. For the never competent patient (newborn or retarded), he outlined a surrogate or proxy arrangement (via family, friend, legal guardian, durable power of attorney, or, in the last resort, physician) and the conditions for a morally valid act by such a proxy or surrogate (he or she must be competent, must know the patient and his values, and there should be no conflict of interest or serious emotional conflict).

Within a pluralistic society and a system of medical care ethics, based on the principles of Autonomy and Beneficence, conflicts are bound to arise—between patient/surrogate, doctor, family, and healthcare team members—as to what is in the best interests of the patient. Hence, various mechanisms must be available for negotiation, consultation and resolution of conflicts—including ethics committees and, in the last resort, courts of law.

At the bedside, the principle of Beneficence is called into play in the face of a host of dilemmas. Beneficence dictates that the effectiveness of an available treatment be weighed against its benefit to the patient. Many treatments may not be beneficial— e.g., an effective treatment for pneumonia in a case of advanced malignant disease—and may violate the patient's autonomy if he/she does not wish to be so treated. Conversely, some treatments may put the patient in danger—(e.g., treatment for pain in malignant disease) yet be beneficial. On the question of whether and when to discontinue life-sustaining measures, Beneficence is again the guiding principle. For the patient in a state of total brain death or in a permanent vegetative state, many, if not most, would feel that life-support measures could be discontinued. But the weakest part of medicine since Hippocrates, Pellegrino argues, always has been prognosis. Patients in coma have been known to recover. Beneficence, in Pellegrino's view (others we might add, may invoke the same principle to argue the opposite), sees the danger of ceasing life-support measures. And Beneficence draws attention to the slippery slope of the progressive devaluation of life, as witnessed by the past 10-year history of court decisions in the U.S.–Quinlan (1976), Conroy (1983–1984), and Bouvier (1986): the respirator may be stopped and the nasogastric tube may be removed from a noncomatose patient. It is tantamount to duty for the health professional to assist the competent patient who so wishes to die.

In terminal care ethics, the most hotly-debated issue in the U.S. is that of the withholding of food and fluids. Court decisions have, for the most part, favored the withdrawal of food and fluids when the benefit of the patient (as interpreted by the medical attendants) is not served. Two extremes cited by Pellegrino are the following: In March 1986, the American Medical Association stated that food and fluids should be regarded as treatment, and could be withdrawn as long as one did not deliberately or willfully aim for the death of the patient. At the other extreme, a group under the auspices of the Pontifical Academy of Sciences, in October 1985, drew a distinction between treatment and care; treatment being intervention that is medically indicated, care being ordinary help due to bedridden patients, as well as compassion and the effective and spiritual support due to every human being in danger. For the terminally ill patient in a brain damaged or vegetative state, treatment could be discontinued, but care (including food and fluids) could not. Indeed, "care" must be lavished upon a patient. In practice, argued Dr. Pellegrino, the principle of Beneficence must guide the physician. In cases where food and fluids are excessively burdensome, merely prolonging life (thereby becoming a mode of injury to the patient and a violation of natural law), they may properly be withdrawn.

The foregoing has been presented as an example of a reasoned, cogent approach to some of the problems of terminal care from the point of view of medical ethics. Though such discussion is a phenomenon of recent origin, it is now commonplace and widespread. In 1970, there were a mere half-dozen articles written in English on healthcare law and ethics. By 1980, there were 14 specialty journals devoted to the field. "Medical ethics" as we now know it, has come into existence in large part as a result of the advent of new life-sustaining treatments and technologies, and of the spectacular developments of modern medical science in the last two decades—organ transplants, the artificial heart, test-tube babies and genetic engineering. While William Schroeder and his artificial heart, and the plight of four-year-old Gabriel Bruce, desperately awaiting a new liver, capture and hold the attention of the public as part of our daily entertainment, medical ethicists and their works multiply ever more rapidly.

Medical ethics, then, is part and parcel of the expanding Western medical-industrial complex. As such it belongs to a social milieu in which public dependence on medical care has reached unprecedented heights, while public trust in the medical profession is close to a breakdown.[10] Healthcare litigation in the U.S. has reached an all-time high, due to a crisis of communication. "The doctor of old had fewer surgical successes, but no suits because he had an ongoing relationship with his patients;" analysis of recent malpractice suits in North America reveals not medical incompetence, but failure to simply sit down and talk.[11] In such an environment, medical ethics attempts to humanize the practice of medicine. The irony is that many of the questions raised by medical ethics (witness the aforementioned food and fluid controversy) serve only to obscure the real issue at stake— the relationship between doctor and patient.

This is not to deny the need for medical ethics. There are now so many things we *can* do—from sustaining severely handicapped newborns to resuscitating the senile dying—that question arises whether we *ought* always to be doing them. The choices that have to be made are often tragic ones of good vs. good (e.g., life vs. quality of life).[12] Careful attempts to clarify such ethical issues must surely benefit those called upon to make life-and-death decisions at the bedside. Our point is, rather, that responsible moral decisions do have to be made by doctors, that the fact must not be obscured, and that the context for making such decisions should be that of a close human relationship with patient and family. In this way, many issues can be gently resolved without being raised to the status of "issues."

In fairness to Dr. Pellegrino, it should be pointed out that a compassionate relationship is, by implication, the silent premise of his ethical system. However, such a premise cannot be assumed to be a universal *sine qua non* at the bedside. Here the situation is further complicated by the fact that responsibility for the individual patient is increasingly fragmented between more and more specialists, having less and less contact with the patient.

The Doctor-Patient Relationship

In this paper we shall argue that the basic issue at stake in the appropriate care of the terminally ill is the doctor-patient relationship. Further, we shall argue that if four "cardinal principles" are to be invoked, they might just as well be the traditional four cardinal virtues. This ethical scheme, in use for many centuries, has in our day fallen into general disuse. Its practical application to the care of the terminally ill has, to our knowledge, never been considered. Yet, its usefulness within the context of the doctor-patient dialogue may readily be appreciated.

In the Middle Ages, this approach was so commonplace that it apparently was not considered necessary to enunciate it with regard to the care of the sick. However, a 15th-century French treatise, *Livre de la vie active*, written by the overseer of the Hôtel-Dieu, a large hospital in Paris, is an exception.[13] The work is a treatise on the active, as distinct from the contemplative, life, which used the service and administration of the Hôtel-Dieu by way of illustration. It provides a vivid glimpse of the practical ethics of the health-care system of that long lost world. In a striking illumination, seven patients in various states of malaise, apparently naked but for their nightcaps, lie tucked up in four beds. At the foot of each bed stands a nun in dark habit, accompanied by two or three small assistant novices in white. Each nun bears on her habit the name of the virtue which she represents, and holds in her hand the symbol by which she ministers to the suffering human beings in her care: prudence (the rod), temperance (the bit), fortitude (the tower), justice (the scales). (See Figure 9-1.)

In the classical scholastic order of things the four cardinal virtues—prudence, justice, fortitude and temperance—took their place after the three theological virtues: faith, hope and charity. Charity was regarded as the foundation and root of every other virtue. And thus, in the care of the sick the necessary virtues might be depicted as shown in Figure 9-2.

In an age when life was "nasty, brutish and short," when human beings lived in full and open awareness of their terminal condition, such was considered fundamental to the appropriate medical care of the terminally ill. If for no other reason it is deserving of our respect and consideration.

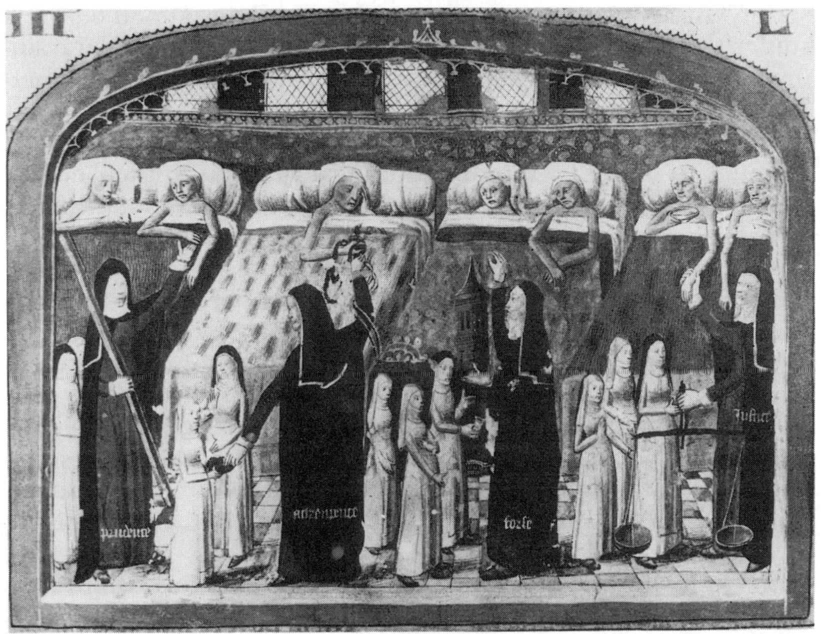

Figure 9-1

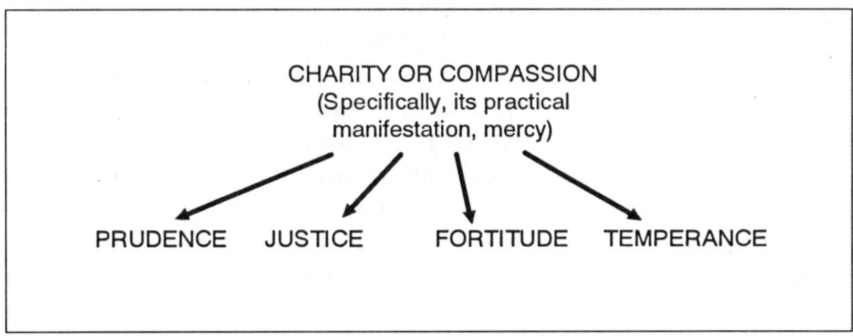

Figure 9-2

It should be stated at the outset that the ideal of care that we are proofing here goes against current moral trends—those of a society which is daily moving deeper and deeper into a value system based on a philosophy of relativism and individual functionalism. The problem is this: The physician is largely a reflection of society. Basic human character traits are well-developed before a student enters medical school. And no amount of medical training can convert a fundamentally self-centered and egotistic person into a humanitarian. "The crisis of humane medicine," it has been said, "is the result of the failure of secular democratic societies to inculcate moral and ethical values into their educational systems."[14] In such a milieu, while there is much talk of moral values and of medical ethics, genuine morality and ethical conduct may remain curiously elusive, for the hallmark of genuine morality is more than a legalistic and impersonal exercise—"justice" or "beneficence" put into action stage by stage. Genuine morality requires personal commitment and spontaneous compassion between human beings. Persons who live life in this way—the doctor or nurse who acts in this way—do so at risk to themselves. Yet, the result may well be a more liberating personal autonomy and authenticity than that which is commonly taken for granted.[15] In this sense "doctor autonomy" is as much an issue at stake as "patient autonomy."

In exploring the moral dimensions of the doctor-patient relationship, one recent work stands as a landmark: Jay Katz, (Professor of Law and Psychoanalysis at Yale) in *The Silent World of Doctor and Patient,* has shown how the legal doctrine of informed consent could and should govern the relationship between physician and patient. Examining the psychological complexities of the doctor-patient interaction, he advocates a change from paternalism to an egalitarian relationship, from one-way to two-way trust, from blind trust to earned trust, from one-sided to shared decision-making. Trust presupposes intimacy. Intimacy cannot exist with deception. Deception exists when we refuse to share our uncertainty with the other person. But when both feel free to share their uncertainty, intimacy is possible and trust is earned. Such things cannot be achieved without cost. "If doctors can learn," Katz argues,

> and in turn teach their patients, that it is possible to sit down and reason together about the most important personal anxieties and fears that illness and its treatment engenders, then they could also point the way to living life, not by submission but by mutual respect, with careful attentiveness to one's own and the other's rationalities and irrationalities.[16]

"Mutual respect" and "careful attentiveness," we shall argue, are synonymous with compassion in action (i.e., mercy). What we propose then is not a set of moral rules, but rather a relationship—a genuine sharing of the self—in the context of which the four cardinal virtues may be taken as guides to appropriate action.

The kind of doctor-patient relationship that we are proposing here, based on compassion in action, is becoming imperative for many reasons, scientific no less than humanitarian. It is increasingly recognized that 20th-century medicine is experiencing a metaphysical crisis. The distinction between mind and body, which came into being at the end of the Middle Ages, was fully articulated by Descartes in the 17th century, and which has dominated modern science until the 20th century, lies at the root of this crisis.[17] While the Cartesian view has been drastically undermined by the discoveries of modern physics (that energy and consciousness, mind and matter, are interdependent, that the world cannot be understood apart from the mind of the observer—that we ourselves are part of the field of energies which we observe, and, hence, that science can never be objective), nevertheless, it remains the basis of the current biomedical model. In the Cartesian paradigm, the patient is viewed as a passive, physiological mechanism, an "object-body." Hence, he or she must rely on outside forces for cure—on a doctor who knows how to fix the mechanism, and on technological intervention of one sort or another—physical (surgery or radiation) or chemical (drugs). Such a paradigm directs attention toward curing the body rather than healing the person, treating the disease rather than the patient. Its dehumanizing effects are only too well-known, yet its principles are thoroughly ingrained in our culture. Increasingly, however, as the narrow conceptual basis of this biomedical model is recognized, so it becomes evident that many subtle, less tangible factors—the emotional state of the patient, the patient's attitude toward his illness, the quality of the therapeutic alliance of the doctor and patient—are fundamental both in diagnosis and prognosis. These things are not new. The 19th-century physician had never heard of the special theory of relativity, nor of Heisenberg's uncertainty principle. But he acted on the assumption that his patients were changed, physically, by his bedside manner.[18] The phenomenon was observed even further by Hippocrates when he remarked, "Some patients, though conscious that their condition is perilous, recover their health simply through their contentment with the goodness of the physician."

Attuned to the mood of modern physics as it may be, the kind of doctor-patient relationship that we are advocating is not attuned to the mood of our society as a whole. Loneliness, habitual isolation, it seems, is indigenous to our culture. And it is increasingly clear that chronic loneliness, lack of human intimacy, lack of companionship or the sudden loss of it, are significant contributors to some of the most serious diseases from which we suffer.[19] For this reason, genuine, close doctor-patient relationships, while more than ever imperative, are far from normal in our culture. This being said, we may now proceed to our exploration of the doctor-patient relationship.

Charity (*mutual respect and careful attentiveness*)

In the face of imminent death, the Cartesian "object-body" biomedical model is unhelpful. When all has been done to ease the dying patient's passage, the caregiver has nothing to offer but himself. For this reason, over the past decade or so, the medical specialty of palliative care has moved ahead of other specialties in articulating (in a growing body of literature) a new kind of approach—one in which the therapeutic alliance of patient-caregiver has been intimately explored, often with great subtlety and sensitivity. The spirit of this new literature is typified by the opening sentence of a recent work in this genre:

> A recurrent theme of this book is the importance of emotional accessibility, the art of being fully present to another human being. Present, not only as an expert in the physiologic nuances of life-threatening illness and treatment, but as a willing companion.[20]

In the brief space available to us here we shall indicate, drawing on the work of some of the most skilled clinicians (those who have attempted to be fully present to the dying patient and to enter into and share his reality) what, in our and their experience, are most commonly perceived (by means of compassion and careful attentiveness) to be the deepest needs of the dying patient.

Four major areas of need identified by the psychiatrist Colin Murray Parkes, are: 1) Physical (need for pain relief), 2) Cognitive (need for information), 3) Affective (need for human closeness) and 4) Spiritual (need for God). All terminally ill patients, he argues, are forced to undergo great changes in their lives. Their world will never be the same again. Countless assumptions, structures of meaning built up over years, suddenly collapse. At a time when security is most needed, the terminally ill patient is beset by interior chaos. Parkes has articulated a theory of psycho-social transitions, which embrace all four of these dimensions. Psycho-social transitions, life changes whose magnitude we are unable, in a short time, to take in or cope with, are characterized in the four areas mentioned above, by: pain (physical and mental), cognitive confusion, intense emotions (pining, anger, bewilderment), and spiritual perplexity, as the meanings of life are shattered. Each must be articulated and shared so that patient and family may pass through the transitions, re-learn their world and find new reasons for living and dying.[21]

When the terminally ill person's internal model of the world, built up from all his previous life experiences, is suddenly shattered, the sense of loss may be overwhelming. Sourkes distinguishes three kinds of loss:[22]

1) Loss of control—of his body, his emotions, of life itself. Paradoxically, this sense of loss of control is usually worsened in the hospital situation, where individual autonomy is given very low priority. (In fact, as the hospice movement has demonstrated, much can be done to support the patient's sense of control.)

2) Loss of identity—"Who am I?" "What is left of me now?" With an altered body image, the patient fears the reactions of others in the face of changes in his appearance. Less visible changes (e.g., in sexuality), may be devastating. His fear is of being defined exclusively in terms of his illness. (When the patient's sense of identity falters, ongoing support and affection from the family and caregiver are crucial.)

3) Loss of relationships—An aspect of human behavior frequently observed when a person is known to be dying, is avoidance or emotional withdrawal on the part of those around. The phenomenon has been repeatedly observed among healthcare professionals, family and friends. It has been called "bereavement of the dying."[23] Struggling with his own disorientation and anticipatory grief in the face of multiple losses—of self, of loved ones, of all that has been important in his life, the patient, with a heightened sense of being alone in the face of the unknown, reaches out for assurance that he will not be abandoned, for love and companionship. In the hospital situation such loneliness is generally intensified, accentuating the suffering of the dying person. In brief, the patient's pain in terminal illness—especially cancer—is the suffering of the whole person, bodily and spiritual, suffering which Saunders terms "total pain."

Having perceived some of the needs of the dying person, we move now to ask what can be done to meet those needs. What is the appropriate treatment under such circumstances?

Weisman has suggested that an "appropriate death" is one we might choose, had we a choice. It is marked by "an absence of suffering, preservation of important relationships, an interval for anticipatory grief, relief of remaining conflicts, belief in timeliness, exercise of feasible options and activities, and consistency with physical limitations, all within the scope of one's ego ideal." It is, in sum, "the final version of an informed consent," in which the patient is enabled to die with dignity, perhaps with greater self-esteem than was known during life. Through realization of his needs, the person remains fully a person as he approaches death, in practice yielding autonomy in decision-making to others, in order to ease his final passage and assure "safe conduct."[24] Such, briefly, is an "appropriate death," a concept which has gained wide acceptance throughout the literature of terminal care.

If an appropriate death is one which respects the humanity and autonomy of the patient, then an appropriate treatment is one which does likewise. Many skilled clinicians, not least Cicely Saunders,[25] have discussed the question of "appropriate treatment" from this point of view. Much has been said about what can be done to support the humanity and autonomy of the patient, both by sensitive, compassionate care, and competent clinical management. Our purpose here is not to retrace the steps of others whose work we could not emulate, rather, it is simply to suggest a new and different dimension to the problem.

If appropriate medical care means that the doctor must *care* for the patient in the fullest sense of the word (i.e., with full attentiveness to the patient as a person) and if this kind of care depends on the quality of the doctor-patient relationship, then appropriate medical care depends on nothing more or less than what the doctor is like as a human being. Or, to put it another way, it is not something which the doctor *does to* the patient. It is, rather, something which springs from the very essence of what he *is*.

What we are proposing then, is not the replacement of one set of ethical principles with another—Patient autonomy, Beneficence, Non-maleficence and Justice, by Prudence, Justice, Fortitude and Temperance—but rather, the nurturing of a dynamic relationship between doctor and patient, within which the four cardinal virtues may serve simply as guides to appropriate action. Most of what we are saying has already been said, in one way or another. And yet it has not. For what we are attempting to do here is to turn the conventional approach inside-out. We are less concerned with what is "appropriate" in this or that situation than with what is the underlying attitude of the doctor toward himself and his patient. When that is fully human the action which flows from the doctor will be fully appropriate.

Finally, lest it be thought that we are advocating human interaction as a substitute for competent medical care, we hasten to point out that Prudence, Justice, Fortitude and Temperance are just as applicable to the clinical realities of the bedside situation as to the emotional-spiritual ones. Mount has drawn attention to the fact that in North American hospice programs clinical skills—charting, history taking, physical examination—often have been insufficient, with inadequate knowledge of pharmacology, pharmacokinetics, neurology, medical oncology and internal medicine. But, he points out, medical incompetence under the guise of high motivation is still medical incompetence; the foundation of whole-person medical care is excellence in *physical* care (here symptom control).[26] With this we would concur, stressing that Prudence, Justice, Fortitude and Temperance embrace every aspect of care in a non-dualistic whole.

1. Prudence: is a steady disposition of practical reason to right action. It has two aspects—one concerned with gathering knowledge, and with establishing a yardstick, the other concerned with evaluation, decision and command. It is the readiness to judge soundly and to act rightly, and as such, is the mother of the other virtues.[27]

In the care of the terminally ill, prudence is called for from the outset. In the question of truth-telling, the ethical maxim *primum non nocere* is part and parcel of this virtue. Over the past 20 years, doctors appear to have to become more inclined to tell cancer patients the truth of their diagnosis, though in some places (e.g., South American countries) the conspiracy of silence is still the rule rather than the exception. Telling the truth of a fatal diagnosis may be regarded as an ethical dilemma—"Should the doctor tell?" As Hinton points out, the question, "Should the doctor tell?" tends to imply that the doctor knows all, and the patient nothing, about the approaching death.[28] In practice, the basic principle of charity (the underlying relation of mutual respect and careful attentiveness) will guide the physician through an ongoing dialogue with the patient toward the most prudent course of action.

The patient has a right to know and a right not to know. In fact, less than three-fourths of patients want to know.[29] With the current trend towards open awareness, many doctors see it as their duty to tell all. But total candor may be overwhelming, if not devastating, to the patient who is not ready to hear. It is important, therefore, that the patient be given the opportunity to control the information he is given. As Saunders puts it, "The real question is not, 'What do you tell your patients?' but rather, 'What do you let your patients tell you?'"[30] Careful attention is needed to the amount of information imparted and the patient's ability to receive it. In this way, the patient has time to accommodate himself in various ways—one of which is by worrying. Worry, Parkes points out, is a way of preparing a possible world that enables us, if our fears are realized, to cope more effectively with the reality which we have now to enter. In situations where information needs to be communicated, it is prudent to begin by finding out how much the recipient knows, or thinks he knows, about his condition. The patient can be encouraged to control the input of information by inviting questions: "Have you got any questions?" (In this area doctors often do not invite questions.) The questions which then follow will reveal quite precisely how much the patient is ready to be told.[31] The process is one of dialogue in which the doctor must be prepared to listen and to respond with care to the need which he senses in the patient. In perceiving what the patient wants to reveal of his thoughts and attempting to meet him where he is, we cement the therapeutic alliance. As Parkes has pointed out,

> He may say, 'I am frightened of dying!' and we hastily murmur, 'Yes, I understand,' and change to some more cheerful subject. Yet the dying patient can fear many things, and a more appropriate response may be, 'Are you? Well tell me just what you mean by that.'[32]

When the message is deeply disturbing, and loaded with information which calls for a major psychosocial transition, it is not surprising that there may be difficulties in communication. The simple statement, "The biopsy was positive," may be so overwhelming that the patient may not be able to take it in. Thus, Parkes points out, it takes time and emotional support to break bad news. Our role is simply to sense where the patient is, and help him to tackle each problem on his own terms, in his own time. The question of control is fundamental. Most people are able to monitor their input of information in order to control the rate at which they restructure their internal world and thus avoiding overload. So what appears to be denial may simply be a postponement of one psychosocial transition in favor of another.[33] In such a situation, considerable understanding and prudence in the face of ambiguity is called for in the caregiver. In any event, those who wish to use denial should not be assaulted by truths that they may not be able to cope with.[34]

Prudence, then, is fundamental when it comes to imparting information *to* the terminally ill patient. In recent years, it has become fundamental in imparting information *about* the terminally ill patient. The issue of confidentiality was addressed recently by Margaret Somerville.[35] In the physician-patient relationship, a basic obligation is that all information regarding the patient be kept confidential, though, of necessity, when the harm done by a legal wrong is less than the harm avoided, the legal wrong may be done in order to avoid the greater harm. In the normal terminal care situation, there is implied consent to the sharing of information with other members of the healthcare team for the benefit of the patient. In most cases, there is no risk that the sharing of that information will have any adverse effects for the patient. With the AIDS situation, however, this is no longer the case. Considerable discernment is needed in judging when confidentiality may be breached by reason of a moral duty to warn a third party of potential or actual danger—as, for example, in the case cited by Somerville, of "Dr. Webster" and his patient "John" with AIDS, about to undergo nonelective surgery, also scheduled for dental treatment, with a pregnant wife. Who should Dr. Webster tell—the surgeon? the dentist? the wife?[36]

At the bedside, prudence bears directly on a host of practical problems, most notably, pain control. In the 1960s the control of intractable pain in the cancer patient was revolutionized by the work of Cicely Saunders, who within the context of care for psychosocial and spiritual needs of the patient, introduced individually optimized doses of narcotics at intervals dependent on the kinetics of the drug used, together with carefully selected coanalgesics.[37] Since then, through the hospice movement, the practice of underprescribing (*p.r.n.* or "as required," rather than continuous and preventive) due to fear of addiction or rapid escalation of the effective dose, has been recognized as inappropriate in the terminal care situation. The terminally ill patient in pain presents a dilemma which requires careful judgment on the part of the physician—that of providing adequate analgesia, while not hastening death by depressing vital functions. The reduction of fear and anxiety is basic to pain control. In our experience, local pain trigger or intravenous injections of procaine have proven beneficial in alleviating both fear and pain, while actually stimulating vital functions. Here it should be stressed, the human presence of the giver of the medication is of singular importance. An attitude of quiet confidence and readiness to listen and to engage in unhurried conversation can go a long way toward alleviating the total pain of the terminally ill patient.

In the wider care of the terminally ill patient, within the setting of the family unit, prudence is indispensable. In times of trouble, most families will rally around to provide care, concern and security for their members. In times of psychosocial transition, however, when the members of the family are often under great stress, the reverse may happen. Members of the family may withdraw and avoid real communication, or negative energies may be released between family members. The concerned caregiver has a role to play in expressing that concern and diplomatically facilitating the family in talking about their underlying difficulties.[38]

2. Justice: The strong and firm will to give to each his due.[39] Somerville's recent discussion of the relation between medicine and law is apposite. Medicine focuses on needs (treatment to relieve suffering), while law focuses on rights (the patient has the right to refuse treatment, hence, a possible conflict exists). A person may refuse treatment which the physician considers necessary for his good. In such a situation the possibility for infliction of suffering is enormous. The danger is that of a breach of human rights in the name of doing good. The law's definition of suffering may be closer to reality than that of medicine, for medical intervention may reduce physical suffering, but increase psychological suffering. Unconsented-to interference makes the person feel as though he has lost control over what happens to him.[40]

Refusal of treatment. When the treatment is refused, the result may be increased pain, but because that refusal was respected, decreased suffering. Refusal of treatment is more common in AIDS patients, where the patient has a fairly clear idea of the outcome, than in other forms of terminal illness. Such refusal may be difficult for the healthcare professional to accept, particularly if the patient is a young person, say in their 20s. Nevertheless, the law states that no treatment can be inflicted upon a competent adult without his informed consent (the patient must be treated as a person, not an object). The patient is not obliged to accept medical treatment, even if refusal results in earlier death. And yet, Somerville argues, the refusal situation in itself may be a therapeutic opportunity. For by respecting the patient's refusal of treatment the healthcare professional, despite the fact that he thinks the patient is making a mistake, augments the therapeutic alliance. The issue at stake here is that of the patient's identity as a person. In the stark words of one AIDS patient: "I hope physicians everywhere will remember they are dealing with real people and not with plastic dolls they can manipulate at whim. I am frightened, but not of death. Rather, I am frightened of being helpless."[41]

Acceptance of treatment. A growing body of evidence indicates that patients who do not have information about their treatment experience a sense of helplessness and high anxiety levels. Patients, psychologically prepared for major surgery by being fully informed about the effects of the operation, warned how they should expect to feel afterwards, advised how they could control pain and encouraged to express their own feelings about what they were experiencing, coped better than those given bland reassurance and minimal information. They required less narcotic drugs, ran less risk of postoperative psychoses and recovered more quickly than those who were not prepared in this way.[42] Parkes cites the case of the amputee patient warned before surgery to expect pain in the phantom limb, who when asked, "Did you have any pain in your foot after it was taken off?" replied, "Yes, I was so pleased.... The doctor had told me to expect it to hurt, so I knew that everything was going according to plan."[43] "As the Nazis well understood and demonstrated," says Le Shan,

> meaningless and purposeless torture is much harder for the person to accept and resist than is torture which the subject can place in a coherent frame of reference. A perceived senselessness in the universe weakens our belief that our efforts have validity and point. They appear to be essentially futile. This makes it much harder to continue these efforts, including those of coping with pain and stress.[44]

It would appear, indeed, that a direct relationship exists between the patient's sense of anxiety or sense of lack of control, and the experience of pain. The phenomenon has been copiously documented by Goldberg and his collaborators, who found that physical suffering responds not merely to pharmacological agents for the relief of pain but, often dramatically, to human contact (simple conversation facilitating resolution of emotional conflicts at times proved to be more efficacious than narcotics) and to increased control on the part of the patient.[45] It is clear that while feelings of helplessness and hopelessness can be shown to have an adverse effect on a patient's prognosis, mutual respect on the part of the doctor and patient can be demonstrated to have positive physiological effects. Oncologist Bernard Siegel recalls the following conversation between his mastectomy patient and her nurse the morning after her operation:

"You have no pain," the nurse said to this patient. "You're walking up and down the wards of the hospital, cheering people up, and you're not supposed to be up like that—you just had a mastectomy!" The patient replied, "There's a big difference. Dr. Siegel did what I wanted done. He and I shared. So why should I have pain, and why should I be upset?"[46]

Such an attitude—of responsibility for one's own health, in the belief that one is a full participant in the healing process—has not been fostered by our society or our medical system, tending as they do to reinforce the notion of the patient as a passive recipient of the doctor's attentions, an object-body, rather than an autonomous person.

3. Fortitude: Courage of soul that strengthens and enables one to adopt and adhere to a reasonable course of action when faced with the danger of death or other grave peril.[47]

Since fortitude is the ability to suffer that which violates one's inner equanimity, that which is negative, painful, oppressive or frightening, it is, perhaps, the medical virtue *par excellence.* For those who deal with the terminally ill, fortitude is called for at every turn. This is particularly true for the healthcare professional who is in most immediate contact with the patient and gives 80 percent or more of all care—the nurse. Terminal care is one of the most demanding situations encountered by nurses. Keeping the patient clean, fed and comfortable to the end is not, as a rule, easy or pleasant. And working with the patient's family also can be very stressful. But, in the words of one such nurse:

The dying person wants and needs a caregiver who is calm, confident, matter-of-fact, and unhurried in manner. Such an approach serves as a source of comfort above and beyond the actual assistance that is given by a treatment or procedure. It carries a message of respect and care that is not easily appreciated by people who have never been ill or totally dependent on others for help. It is also difficult to provide day after day because it makes tremendous demands on the nurse's capacities and resources and is psychologically draining because of these demands.[48]

What enables the caregiver to sustain this kind of involvement with people who are seriously ill and dying? The ability called for here—to take emotional risks, to experience deep feelings, to share the reality of patient and family in distress, and to engage in repeated cycles of attachment-loss, can lead to what is commonly termed "emotional burnout." In order to step into the lives of those whose existence is founded on such uncertainty, the caregiver must possess a high tolerance for ambiguity and an inner freedom to flow with the experience without needing to impose a rigid structure.[49] Feifel and others have stressed the caregiver's need to come to terms with her own fears of personal death, without which there is avoidance of open encounter with the dying person. In nursing literature over the past decade, much emphasis has been placed on recognizing and meeting the "Needs of the Dying Patient." An increasing amount of evidence indicates that emphasis needs to be placed on the "Needs of the Nurse who is Nursing the Dying Patient." Experienced nurses have attested to the fact that irrespective of the patient's medical problems, it is only as the nurse is able to come to terms with herself, her own conflicts and anxieties, her negative and "unprofessional" feelings, that she is able truly to enter into the stressful world of another.[50] The terminally ill patient has an acute sense of vision, to which the caregiver's anxieties become transparent. Coming to terms with one's own fears of death would appear to be fundamental in encountering the terminally ill person.

And yet, counters Parkes, how do we know that we have faced up to the reality of our own death until after we are dead? What does matter, in the end, is the kind of commitment that enables the caregiver to "hang in" with those in deep distress—a commitment facilitated by compassion. The fact is that those who care for the dying in the most effective and compassionate way more often than not have a religious commitment of one sort or another. And, thus, we are drawn back to our starting point—to charity—a concept with theological dimensions which lie beyond the scope of this paper—of participation in the divine love.

If fortitude is called for in those who care for the terminally ill, it is needed still more by the terminally ill person himself. Such fortitude cannot but be encouraged and sustained by an authentic caregiver-patient relationship. Open and trusting communication between patient-caregiver and patient-patient (whether in group psychotherapy or otherwise) has been shown to facilitate self-exploration and self-integration, which sometimes results in profound inner growth among the terminally ill.[51] "People who are dying," observes Saunders, "often have a tremendous capacity for meeting, or encountering, because they have put aside the mask that we tend to wear in every day life."[52] The subtle dynamics of this healing process have been described by LeShan, who points out how basic is real "encounter," real human contact, between patient and therapist. If the therapist has reservations about fully meeting the patient, the patient will sense this, and his own reservations about meeting life and meeting himself will be reinforced.[53] Mount has observed that while life-threatening illness carries the potential for great psychological distress, it also may be an unusual opportunity for interior growth, both individually and in relationships. The physician's unique opportunity to act as a catalyst to the growth (if simply to assist patients in identifying "meaning" in their lives, reviewing the things they have created, believed, loved and left behind) is awesome.[54] We would add that if the doctor-patient will act as a catalyst in the doctor's growth—the doctor may come to know himself through the patient's eyes.

4. Temperance: is a virtue by which we are able to achieve a certain moderation with respect to objects which attract us—moderation both of our desire for them and of our sorrow when they are absent. Tranquility of soul is said to belong to all the virtues, but especially to temperance.[55]

While the caregiver and the healthy person may equate "hope" with "life," for the terminally ill patient, the will to stay alive generally diminishes, and the time usually comes when the focus of hope shifts to other goals—hopes for absence of pain, for companionship of family and friends, for a doctor who will not abandon him, for assurance of the welfare of loved ones when he is gone.[56] Quality of life is a highly individual thing. Good quality of life is attained, argues Twycross, when hopes are matched by circumstances.[57]

Temperance comes into focus most sharply in the vexed question of the prolongation of life. The question is a difficult one for the physician, whose art is to preserve life, to cure and keep alive. The key principle here, it would seem, is to avoid futile treatments. As Twycross has pointed out, the question "to treat or not to treat?" is inappropriately formulated. The question should rather be, "what is the appropriate treatment, given this patient's prospects?" Resuscitative measures such as intravenous infusions, blood transfusions, C.P.R., the use of antibiotics, respirators and coronary care units, were intended to help the patient through an acute crisis on the basis of his previous biological prospects. The moribund patient may be offered such a treatment. If it prolongs the distress of dying rather than prolonging or supporting useful life, such treatment would seem inappropriate under the circumstances.[58]

Thus stated, and seen always in the context of mutual respect and careful attentiveness, and of continuing communication with patient and family, what may be turned into a big ethical question—to treat or not to treat—is reduced to less momentous proportions. The doctor does not have a duty, legally or ethically, to prolong life at all costs. In certain circumstances, as Twycross points out, we have to give death a chance, which is not the same as killing the patient. His "two-day rule" is suggested as a practical guide. If the terminally ill patient develops a chest infection and the caregiver is not certain how close he is to death, instead of immediately prescribing antibiotics, he might review the situation tomorrow and the following day. If the patient is much worse, the answer is clear. If the patient is holding his own but troubled by a problem of expectoration, then antibiotics would appear to be indicated.[59]

In the hospital setting the availability of new technology (e.g., respirators), hospital regulations, pressures from hospital bureaucracies and a certain human dynamic among the staff, set into motion a certain momentum making it difficult for the individual caregiver to refrain from using such technology even against his better judgment. And over any decision not to use life-prolonging technology, there hovers what has been called "the brooding presence of medical liability."[60] Fifty years ago, pneumonia was known as "the old man's friend." Hospital regulations now require any patient in an intensive care unit, in coma or otherwise, who contracts pneumonia automatically be treated for it. Under such circumstances, temperance is far from easily sustained. The quandary is well-known, and it arises in a variety of situations, apart from terminal illness—with patients in coma, accident victims and newborn infants with incurable defects. The quiet, gentle death of bygone centuries has been replaced by a long, drawn-out death, so that it would seem that the only way left for a person to die a "good death" (i.e., "euthanasia") is to be killed somehow.[61]

Temperance, the virtue of moderation or right proportion, brings us back to the starting point of this paper, the starting point for a reasonable, balanced medical care of the terminally ill—the realization of our terminal condition, of the brevity and fragility of life, symbolized by the poignant image of the sparrow.

The appropriate medical care of the terminally ill patient is based on a relationship of mutual respect and careful attentiveness between patient and caregiver. This relationship, we have argued, requires the cardinal virtues of prudence, justice, fortitude and temperance for its completeness. Western medical thinking is still dominated by dualism and mechanism, by a modality of thought which separates mind/body, subject/object, doctor/patient. The mechanistic model, however, is slowly but surely disintegrating. It has been shown to be obsolete for the needs of modern physics. It is now also beginning to appear inadequate for the needs of contemporary medicine. In its place is emerging a unified model which expresses dynamic wholeness, an implicate order connecting consciousness and physical reality.[62] In the light of this, prudence, justice, fortitude and temperance, founded in charity, are more than moralistic constructs superimposed on a obsolete mechanistic foundation. They are, rather, states of being, part of an underlying preestablished harmony of the universe in which physical/physiological facts and thought itself cannot ultimately be separated one from the other. The dynamic relationship between patient and caregiver, informed by these qualities of soul, is ultimately a reflection of that order. Its recognition is vital to medicine as a whole—both to its art and its science.

The doctor-patient relationship has, in our day, fallen into neglect. That neglect lies at the heart of the present crisis in medicine, a medicine in which science and art have become separated. Fragmentation, separation and alienation reflect the underlying malaise of our culture. No longer are we able to see life as a whole. If its transcendence escapes us, so, in general, does its transience. And yet, as Mrs. D.Z., aged 88, remarked to her

Toronto doctor: "My mother used to say that we're only here for a visit—we come in through one door and go out through another."

NOTES

1. B. Colgrave and R.A.B. Mynors (eds. and translators), *Bede's Ecclesiastical History of the English People* (Oxford: Clarendon Press, 1969) 183–185.

2. M.J. Arlen, "The Air. The Cold, Bright Charms of Immortality," *The New Yorker,* January 27, 1975, 73–78.

3. A. van Gennep, *The Rites of Passage,* translated by M.B. Vizedom and G.L. Caffee (London: Routledge and Kegan Paul, 1960).

4. P. Laslett, *The World We Have Lost* (London: Methuen, 1965), 103; *World Population Prospects: Estimates and Projections as Assessed in 1982* (United Nations Publications, Sales No.83.XIII.5).

5. P. Laslett, *The World We Have Lost,* 104.

6. D.M. Frame (translator), *The Complete Works of Montaigne* (Stanford, CA.: Stanford University Press, 1943) 236–237.

7. I. Illich, "The Political Uses of Natural Death," in P. Steinfels and R.M. Veatch (eds.), *Death Inside Out. The Hastings Center Report* (New York: Harper and Row, c. 1974, 1975) 25–42, at 39.

8. C.C. Gotay, "Models of Terminal Care: A Review of the Research Literature," *Clinical and Investigative Medicine* 6 (1983) 131–141.

9. R. Twycross, "Decision-Making: What is Appropriate." Communication addressed to a seminar, "Advances in Symptom Control," at the Sixth Congress on Care of the Terminally Ill, Montreal, September 27–October 1, 1986.

10. The rising tide of public disenchantment is witnessed by the press: "'Crude and arrogant behavior' cited in complaints about MDs," *Toronto Star,* 24 July 1986.

11. E. LeBourdais, "Talk is cheap, litigation isn't," *Canadian Doctor,* August 1986, 7–8, at 8.

12. J.E. Thomas, "Good vs. good: 'tragic' choice," *Canadian Doctor,* February 1986, 19–20.

13. MS Archives Assistance Publique, Paris, layette 330, liasse 1438. For extracts from this work, see E. Coyecque, *L'Hôtel-Dieu de Paris au moyen âge,* 2 vols. (Paris: H. Champion, 1889–1891).

14. S.M. Glick, "Humanistic Medicine in a Modern Age," *New England Journal of Medicine* 304 (1981) 1036–1038, at 1038.

15. K.M. Gow, *Yes, Virginia, There is Right and Wrong* (Wheaton, Illinois: Tyndale House, 1985) 64, 84.

16. Jay Katz, *The Silent World of Doctor and Patient* (New York: Free Press, 1986), 226.

17. F. Capra, *The Turning Point. Science, Society, and the Rising Culture* (London: Wildwood House, 1982) Chapter 5; J. Gold, "Cartesian Dualism and the Current Crisis in Medicine—Plea for a Philosophical Approach: Discussion Paper," *Journal of the Royal Society of Medicine* 78 (1985), 663–666.

18. Cf. J.J. Lynch, *The Broken Heart. The Medical Consequences of Loneliness* (New York: Basic Books, 1977,) 197.

19. See Lynch, *The Broken Heart,* and J.J. Lynch, *The Language of the Heart. The Body's Response to Human Dialogue* (New York: Basic Books, 1985).

20. C.A. Garfield (ed.), *Psychosocial Care of the Dying Patient* (New York: McGraw Hill, 1978), 3.

21. C.M. Parkes, "Life Transitions." Address to the third plenary session of the Sixth World Congress on Care of the Terminally Ill.

22. B. Sourkes, "The Deepening Shade...Psychological Aspects of Life-Threatening Illness." Address to the second plenary session of the Sixth World Congress on Care of the Terminally Ill.

23. On "bereavement of the dying" see A.D. Weisman and T.P. Hackett, "Predilection to Death," *Psychosomatic Medicine* 23 (1961), 232–256. On the phenomenon of withdrawal from the dying, see B.G. Glaser and A.L Strauss, *Awareness of Dying* (Chicago: Aldine, 1965); R.A. Kalish, "Social Distance and the Dying," *Community Mental Health Journal* 2 (1966), 152–155. On social isolation and loneliness among dying patients, particularly those hospitalized in acute care settings, see the literature cited by M.V. Zack, "Loneliness: A Concept Relevant to the Care of Dying Persons," in *The Nursing Clinics of North America* 20 (1985), 403–414.

24. A.D. Weisman, "The Psychiatrist and the Inexorable" in H. Feifel (ed.), *New Meanings of Death* (New York: McGraw Hill, 1977), 107–122, at 119.

25. C. Saunders (ed.), "Appropriate Treatment, Appropriate Death," *The Management of Terminal Malignant Disease,* 2nd edition (London: Edward Arnold, 1984), 1–16.

26. B.M. Mount, "Challenges in Palliative Care. Four Clinical Areas that Confront and Challenge Hospice Practitioners," Keynote Address, First Annual American Conference on Hospice Care, June 9–11, 1984, Boston, Massachusetts.

27. Thomas Aquinas, *Summa Theologiae,* Blackfriars edition, 61 vols. (London: Eyre and Spottiswoode, 1964–1981), 2a, 2ae, q.47 ff.

28. J. Hinton, *Dying,* 2nd edition (Harmondsworth, Middlesex: Penguin, 1972), 126.

29. R. Higgs, "On Telling Patients the Truth" in *Moral Dilemmas in Modern Medicine,* M. Lockwood (ed.), (Oxford: Oxford University Press, 1985), 187–202, at 196.

30. C. Saunders, "The Moment of Truth: Care of the Dying Person," in L. Pearson (ed.), *Death and Dying. Current Issues in the Treatment of the Dying Person* (Cleveland, Ohio: Case Western Reserve University, 1969), 49–78, at 59.

31. C.M. Parkes,"Life Transitions," *op. cit.*
32. C.M. Parkes, "Psychological Aspects" in *Management of Terminal Malignant Disease* Saunders (ed.), 43–63, at 46.
33. C.M. Parkes, "Life Transitions," *op. cit.*
34. Some recent brief, sensitive treatments of the question are those of H.P. Hogshead, "The Art of Delivering Bad News" in *Psychosocial Care*, C.A. Garfield (ed.), 128–129, and B.M. Mount, "In the Arena of Death," *Canadian Doctor*, February 1986, 6–8.
35. Margaret Somerville, "AIDS: A Test of the Validity and Viability of Health Care Law and Ethics," Communication addressed to a seminar on AIDS at the Sixth World Congress on Care of the Terminally Ill.
36. *Ibid.*
37. B.M. Mount, "Keynote Address." On pain control, see C. Saunders and M. Baines, *Living with Dying. The Management of Terminal Disease* (Oxford: Oxford University Press, 1983); K.M. Foley and C.E. Inturrisi, *Opoid Analgesics in the Management of Clinical Pain, Advances in Pain Research and Therapy*, vol. 8 (New York: Raven Press, 1986).
38. C.M. Parkes, "Life Transitions," *op.cit.*
39. Thomas Aquinas, *Summa Theologiae*, 2a. 2ae. q.57ff.
40. Margaret Somerville, "AIDS," *op. cit.* On the distinction between pain and suffering, see the fundamental paper of E.J. Cassell, "The Nature of Suffering and the Goals of Medicine," *New England Journal of Medicine* 306 (1982) 639–645.
41. Somerville, "AIDS."
42. C.M. Parkes, "Life Transitions," *op.cit.*
43. *Ibid.*
44. L. LeShan, "The World of the Patient in Severe Pain of Long Duration," *Journal of Chronic Diseases* 17 (1964), 119–126, at 120.
45. I.K. Goldberg, A.H. Kutscher, S. Malitz (eds.), *Pain, Anxiety and Grief. Pharmacotherapeutic Care of the Dying Patient and the Bereaved* (New York: Columbia University Press, 1986).
46. J. Kantor, "Bernie Siegel, M.D. A Yale Surgeon Cuts Through the Medical-Authority Myth," *Whole Life Times*, December 1983, 16–19, at 18.
47. Thomas Aquinas, *Summa Theologiae*, *op. cit.*, 2a, 2ae, q.123f.
48. J. Quint Benoliel,"Nurses and the Human Experience of Dying" in H. Feifel (ed.), *op. cit.*, 123–142.
49. B. Sourkes, "The Deepening Shade," *op. cit.*
50. K.M. Gow, *How Nurses' Emotions Affect Patient Care. Self Studies by Nurses* (New York: Springer, 1982), 293–296. K.M. Gow, 234–235.
51. E. Kübler Ross, *Death. The Final Stage of Growth* (Englewood Cliffs, New Jersey: Prentice-Hall, 1975); S.P. Lindenberg, *Group Psychotherapy with People who are Dying* (Springfield, Illinois: Charles C. Thomas, 1983).
52. C. Saunders, "The Moment of Truth," *op. cit.* 78.

53. L. LeShan, "Psychotherapy and the Dying Patient" in L. Pearson (ed.), *Death and Dying op. cit.*, 28–48, at 35.
54. B.M. Mount, "The Ultimate Meaning," *Canadian Doctor*, March 1986, 17–19, at 19.
55. Thomas Aquinas, *Summa Theologiae, op. cit.*, 2a, 2ae, q.141 ff.
56. B.M. Mount, "The ultimate meaning," *op. cit.*, 19.
57. R. Twycross, "Decision-Making: What is Appropriate," *op. cit.*
58. *Ibid.*
59. *Ibid.*
60. J. Ladd (ed.), *Ethical Issues Relating to Life and Death* (New York: Oxford University Press, 1979), 5.
61. *Ibid.*, 4.
62. L. Dossey, *Space, Time and Medicine* (Boston: Shambhala, 1982).

TEN

The RIGHT to DIE

Patrick Nowell Smith

Do we have a right to die and in a manner of our own choosing? That this question is being more and more urgently asked is due to two changes—technological and social—that have occurred in our lifetime. Modern medical technology has virtually eliminated the main killer diseases of the past; most importantly, the introduction of antibiotics has made possible the prevention and cure of pneumonia, a disease that used to be called "the dying man's friend." Human beings can be kept biologically alive, though unconscious, almost indefinitely.

As for the social change, before World War I, there could hardly have been an adult who had never watched over a parent, baby, child, neighbor, or friend and seen them die. In short, death was familiar. And *accepted.* Sad, to be sure, often very sad indeed, but nonetheless accepted as part of the natural order of things, talked about openly, and frequently treated in literature. All that has changed. Apart from those professionally concerned, few of us have seen a corpse unless it was laid out for viewing. Most of us will die in an institution. Death has replaced sex as the unmentionable topic.

Euthanasia is commonly divided into "active" (killing) and "passive" (letting die), a distinction to be challenged later. It is also divided into "voluntary," i.e., at the request or with the consent of the person and "involuntary," without such consent.

The legal position in the United Kingdom is simple. Until 1961, suicide always had been a Common Law crime and aiding suicide was, therefore, automatically a crime as well. The successful suicide could not, of course, be prosecuted. But he suffered certain disabilities, such as forfeiture of goods; and an unsuccessful suicide could be prosecuted. By 1961, these practices had fallen into disuse, and when the crime of suicide was formally abolished, a new statutory offense of aiding suicide was introduced (except in Scotland), carrying a maximum penalty of 14 years. Active euthanasia was always murder and still is. So much for the law on paper, which is pretty much the same in all Common Law jurisdictions.

However, this severity towards mercykilling and aiding suicide is in practice greatly mitigated by the wide powers of sentencing which our legal system accords to judges. If a doctor allows a grossly deformed baby to die, he will be discharged if he can show that his decision not to treat the baby was standard medical practice, and there must be many cases which are not even prosecuted. Also, where the motivation is clearly compassionate, judges usually impose a very light sentence or none at all.

Since the methods most of us would choose to commit suicide require the cooperation of others and that cooperation is illegal, it is clear that we have, at best, a very restricted *legal* right to die at a time and manner of our own choosing. Whether or not we have a *moral* right, which ought to be acknowledged by the law, will depend on the type of moral theory we take as a starting point. On a theory which starts with the concept of individual rights, we have a right to do anything we like, provided there are no good reasons for prohibiting what we want to do, for example, that it infringes the equal right of another. The countervailing reasons can be divided into the religious, the moral and the practical.

Of the religious reasons, little need be said. It is argued that we are not absolute owners of our lives, but hold them in trust from a God who gave them to us, so that the times of our dying should be chosen, not by us, but by God. But whatever the theoretical merits of this argument, religious freedom is deeply embedded in our society that it would be wrong to base any prohibition solely on the grounds that others have a religious objection to what we propose to do.

210

For a rights theorist, the negative right to life, the right not to be killed, is the most fundamental of all rights. When rights are listed, it always comes first, for the very good reason that to deprive someone of life is to deprive him at one blow of all his rights, of all possibilities of earthly enjoyment. But if we grant, as no doubt we all do, that everyone has this negative right to life, it follows at once that we have a right to choose to die. For it is a feature of all rights that they can be invoked or not *at the option of the right-holder*. If you owe me ten dollars, I have a right to demand and get ten dollars from you. But I have no *duty* to require payment; I am at liberty, if I so choose, to waive my right, in this example to forgive the debt. Similarly, the correlative of my right to life is the duty that falls on you not to kill me; but I can release you from this duty by requesting you to kill me or giving my consent. To deny this is to confuse the right to life with a duty, if there is one, to go on living.

And in special circumstances, there may be such a duty. For example, if a person is the sole breadwinner of a family and has no life insurance it may well be his or her duty to struggle on against the desire to die. For some few of us, perhaps some larger loyalty, even the national interest might require us to forego our right to die; but such considerations are rare and not likely to figure in the type of case that leads people to call for changes in the law on euthanasia and aiding suicide, that of people who either from incurable disease or from senility are unlikely to contribute substantially to the good of others.

A large majority of the people who join voluntary euthanasia societies are people in their 60s and 70s who are still enjoying life but do not like what they see in front of them in a society in which more than three-quarters of us will die in institutions. They do not ask for the various guides to self-deliverance issued by some of these societies because they want to use the information now, but because they want the security of knowing that, in the words of John Donne, the keys of their prisonhouse are in their own hands. The following letter sent to the Canadian society *Dying with Dignity* is typical:

I am 79 years of age, in relatively vigorous health and constantly amused with life while it lasts. But I saw my mother and my father, years apart,

> in the same chronic care hospital suffering helplessly for months when they might have been quietly released; and this makes me dread a similar fate unless the law is changed so that one can choose, if still able, to slip away in dignity from the inhumane methods many hospitals employ today to keep one from dying a natural death.

Inevitably, some people will be sad when a person dies; but that sadness is coming to them anyway, and should be diminished rather than increased by the thought that the person they loved died as he or she wished to die.

But what if there is no one willing to kill me or to help me to die? What then happens to my right to choose death? This objection can be met by pointing out that the right to life and its corollary, the right to die, are only negative rights. My right to life imposes on you a duty not to kill me without my consent, but it imposes no duty on you to keep me alive, though you may for other reasons have such a duty. The same is true of the right to die. Supporters of voluntary euthanasia are not asking for Death on Demand. They are not asking that anyone be saddled with a duty to kill someone who asks for death. They assert only that neither a person who asks for help in dying nor a person, if there is one, who is willing to give such help is committing a moral wrong; and they claim that this moral position should be reflected in our criminal law.

Rights-based theories are not the only moral theories. If we look at the question from the point of view of the main rival theory, Utilitarianism, we get the same result. The Utilitarian judges the morality of an action by assessing the good and evil consequences, for the agent and all others concerned, of either doing the action or not doing it. Obviously, such calculations are not easy; but they are not always impossible. *Ex hypothesi* the person whose life or death is at issue has, when he asks for death, come to the conclusion that, for himself, dying is better than staying alive. He may be mistaken, but in many cases this is most unlikely, and in any case he is the best judge of his own interests. As for the interests of others, his choosing to die will be morally right so long as the benefit his remaining alive would confer on them is less than the burden it would place on them and on himself.

What, now, of the practical arguments: arguments to the effect that even if the moral admissibility of voluntary euthanasia were conceded, proposals to change the law would run into insuperable difficulties? First, no proposal to change the law has any chance of success unless it has the support of the medical profession which, it is said, it will never have. "Doctors vary in their approach to passive euthanasia, but the profession condemns legalized active voluntary euthanasia." [1] Nevertheless, there are physicians who practice it, though it is impossible to find out how many do so since they will not admit doing so in public. In the present state of British law such an admission would be a confession of murder.

Voluntary, active euthanasia is practiced openly in Holland, where there are between 5,000 and 6,000 cases a year.[2] The procedure starts with an application by the patient. A team is then formed, consisting always of a doctor and a nurse, a pastor, if the patient asks for one, and others as appropriate.[3] The team discusses the application with the patient and either grants or refuses it. Dr. Pieter Admiraal, a leading proponent of the practice, was convicted some years ago of aiding suicide but was discharged on the grounds that his actions were medically necessary. "What made Dr. Admiraal's actions acceptable were (1) the patient's voluntary and spontaneous requests; (2) the rational and 'durable' nature of the requests; (3) the presence of unacceptable and 'endless' suffering, and (4) Dr. Admiraal's consultation with his colleagues." [4] If the consensus of medical opinion can change in Holland, it could change in other countries, too.

The second type of practical objection comes from the lawyers since the legal profession, like the medical, is on the whole opposed to active euthanasia and aiding suicide. Two years ago, the Law Reform Commission of Canada produced a report on *Euthanasia, Suicide and Cessation of Treatment* which recommended no change in the law other than a clarification of the patient's right to refuse treatment. One of the Commission's arguments for this conservative stance was to the effect that the law in action is much less harsh than the law on paper:

> Our legal system has internal mechanisms which offset the apparent harshness of the law. It is *possible* that in *some* circumstances the accused would be allowed to plead guilty to a lesser charge...Finally in *truly exceptional circumstances*, the authorities already have it within their discretion to decide not to prosecute.[5]

But this is cold comfort, indeed, since the circumstances in which euthanasia or help in committing suicide would be appropriate are, even now, not "truly exceptional;" and as the population ages and the power of medical technology to keep people "alive" increases, they are likely to become even more common.

Many doctors and paramedics are humane; they would like to put an end to suffering they know to be helpless. They are also, on the whole, law-abiding people, and they have a special need to be careful of their reputations. That they are less inclined than they used to be to follow their humane inclinations is due to fear of possible prosecution and, especially in the United States, of malpractice suits if they do not pull out all the stops to keep a patient alive. It is less than fair to say to them, as the Commission in effect does, "what you are doing is against the law, but we *may* turn a blind eye."

The Commission's second line of argument was that any relaxation of the law could lead to mistakes and to serious abuses. This is a serious argument and will be examined later, but it is surprising that the Commission did not consider the possibility of building into a more liberal law safeguards against abuse. Perhaps the reason for this omission was that it relied most heavily on its third line of argument, that relaxation of the law would be "morally unacceptable to the majority of the Canadian people."[6] But is it? This is not a moral question, but a question of empirical fact, and the Commission should surely have produced some evidence for their opinion. It not only cited no evidence, it ignored such evidence as there is. In 1968, the Canadian Institute for Public Opinion (Gallup Poll) asked the following narrowly worded question:

> When a person has an incurable disease that causes great suffering, do you or do you not think that competent doctors should be allowed by law to end the patient's life through mercy killing, if the patient has made a formal request in writing.

In 1968, 45 percent of the firm answers were "Yes," 43 percent were "No." In 1974, the proportions were 55 percent to 35 percent. By 1978, the Yes's outnumbered the No's by more than 2-to-1, and this figure was confirmed in 1984. In Britain, a similarly worded poll in 1969 showed 51 percent of the population in favor of active voluntary euthanasia. By 1976, the proportion had increased to 69 percent; in 1985, it was 72 percent. In the United States the trend is similar, though the proportion of favorable replies is lower. In 1973, the Harris Poll showed only 37 percent in favor; by January 1985, it had reached 61 percent.[7]

The disparity between legal and public thinking also can be illustrated by many cases in which a decision of a court has been criticized in editorials even of newspapers of a generally conservative complexion. One example must suffice. In December 1984, an 84-year-old lady, who had many reasons for ending her life, tried to commit suicide by taking a lethal drug. She had a legal right to do so, but fearful that the attempt might not be successful, she asked a friend, Mrs. Charlotte Hough, to sit with her and to place a plastic bag over her head after she had lost consciousness. Mrs. Hough did what she was asked and reported her action to the police. She was initially charged with murder, but because of the uncertainty as to whether the old lady's death was due to the drugs or to the plastic bag, she was charged with attempted murder. She pleaded guilty and was sentenced to nine months imprisonment, a sentence upheld on appeal.[8] The Judge said that although he had the greatest sympathy for Mrs. Hough, a prison sentence was necessary to uphold the law. On this, *The Sunday Times* commented:

> What is often morally right in this sensitive area remains legally incorrect because, as a nation, we tend to sweep discussion of death under the carpet. In 1976, Baroness Wootton introduced a bill into the House of Lords which would have brought a modicum of good sense and regulation to the subject of euthanasia. But it was not supported. As a result, uncounted numbers of people kept alive by medical science, often die without dignity...Mrs. Hough's crime was compassion and it served to underline once more the need for better legislation governing voluntary euthanasia and the dangers of being without it. People should be allowed to die on their own terms and, as Barbara Wootton once wrote, "not those of nature's cruelty or doctors" ingenuity.[9]

The third type of practical objection arises from the possibility that mistakes will be made and abuses will occur. It would be a pity if someone were to choose death when a cure for his condition was just around the corner. As it stands, this objection is based on a misunderstanding of the nature of biomedical research. The time that elapses between someone's thinking of a new drug or a new application of a known drug and its actual availability is to be measured, not in weeks or months, but in years. So, if there is really a new treatment likely to be available soon, that fact will be known, and the patient should be told what medical treatment can do for him now or in the near future and left to make a choice as to whether or not to hang on and hope for the best. New cures apart, there certainly have been cases of most remarkable and unexpected recovery; so it may well be true that some people who choose death would have recovered to lead meaningful lives. But such cases must, if we can have any faith in medical science, be very rare indeed, and, from the very nature of choice, we can never know if one has occurred. So again the choice should be left to the patient.

The possibility that a more liberal law might be abused is a much more serious objection. How can we be sure that when a patient chooses death the choice is *fully voluntary*? Obviously, this opens one of the most notorious cans of worms in the history of philosophy. Aristotle defined a voluntary action as one not done under compulsion or due to certain types of ignorance,[10] and no one has been able to improve significantly on that definition. The immediate problem is what counts as compulsion. Subtle pressures that would not amount to coercion in law might be put on old people to sign their own death warrants, for example, by greedy heirs who want to inherit, or by family members who might want to get the old person off their backs. Senility, even without the aid of high technology, can last quite a long time and people who need constant care can be a great nuisance. In such a situation, it is possible to insinuate that the old person really has a duty to get out of the way, though it should be noted in passing that in the majority of cases the pressure is the other way.

A more liberal law to mitigate the uncertainties and inhumanity of our current laws is urgently needed, but the problem of building into such a law adequate safeguards against abuse is one, not for philosophers, but for lawyers. For the law has great experience in dealing with problems of coercion and consent in other areas. For example, the validity of a contract may depend on whether the parties freely consented to its terms and in many crimes the guilt of the accused depends on whether or not he intended of his own free will to commit the forbidden act. So we might, for example, insist that possible sources of coercion be fully investigated, that the would-be suicide has been fully informed of the options, and that his will has been expressed several times over a stipulated period. In the Dutch system the most serious abuses, coercion and fraud, are virtually eliminated since active voluntary euthanasia is practiced openly, only in hospitals, and after consultations so thorough that there can be no reasonable doubt that the patient's request is uncoerced, reasonable and durable.

Passive euthanasia (letting one die), whether voluntary or not, seems now to be generally accepted except, perhaps, in the United States where it is still condemned by Right to Life groups. But, while most religious leaders, doctors and lawyers allow it to be morally permissible, they still regard active euthanasia as morally wrong. Their standard morality can be summed up in Clough's often quoted words, "Thou shalt not kill, but needst not strive officiously to keep alive." But what, if any, is the difference?

There is certainly a *conceptual* difference between killing and letting die. A lifeguard who holds a child's head under water till he drowns certainly kills the child; a lifeguard who sits on the bank watching the child drown certainly does not. He lets the child die. But is there any *morally relevant* difference between these two cases? Is not the lifeguard in the second case just as culpable, just as responsible for the death of the child as the lifeguard in the first case? The law has long accepted the principle that acts of omission can be just as criminal as acts of commission and popular morality accepts that they can be just as reprehensible.

So causing death is still causing death, whether the act is one of killing or merely of letting die when one could intervene to save life. If a baby is born with Tay-Sachs disease or anencephalic, it is routine practice to prescribe "nursing care only;" specifically, antibiotics are not given, and if the baby dies, this is thought of as a merciful dispensation of Providence. But in this sort of case the physician does not stand powerlessly by; he has the ability and the opportunity to prevent the death and is fully aware of the fact that, if he intervened, the baby would live, even if only for a little while. In such a case the physician, by refraining from intervention, intentionally and deliberately causes the baby's death, and there is no moral difference in favor of causing death by deliberate non-intervention over causing death by a positive act. If the former is morally permissible, as it is agreed to be, so, too, is the latter; on this point the standard morality is confused. Moreover, if pain is taken into account, a moral difference can be seen in favor of killing the baby. For assuming it to be conscious at all, its suffering is less.

In spite of this, the medical profession is extremely reluctant to accept the morality of active euthanasia, and this is understandable since physicians are by training dedicated to the preservation of life. But the fundamental principle of medical ethics always has been that a physician should act in the best interest of his patient, and it is not always in the best interest of a patient to stay alive. That this is so has recently been recognized by two eminent bodies, the World Medical Assembly[11] and the United States President's Commission for the Study of Ethical Problems in Medicine and Biomedical and Behavioral Research.[12] Both of these bodies advocate passive euthanasia in some cases as preferable to the use of "extraordinary" measures to keep a person alive. What neither of them asks, however, is whether letting a person die, even with the best possible care, really is in his or her best interest.

The question of what is in a person's best interest is not an easy one to answer and the World Medical Assembly did not attempt to answer it; but the President's Commission did.

> In its report "Deciding to Forego Life Sustaining," the Commission says that all patients have an interest in well-being and that, in addition to this, normal adult or competent patients also have an interest in self-determination...In other words, seriously disabled infants should, according to the Commission, not have their lives sustained if their lives are likely to contain more suffering and frustrated desires than happiness and satisfactions.[13]

In line with the Commission's thinking, the United States Surgeon General recommended that an infant who cannot be nourished orally "should not be put on hyperalimentation for a year and a half...but should be provided with a bed and food by mouth knowing that it was not going to be nutritious" and, thus, allowed to die.[14] But once it has been decided that it is better for the baby to die than to be kept alive by "extraordinary" means, would it not be in his best interest to die quickly and painlessly rather than slowly and perhaps painfully?

> In one recently publicized case, an 85-year-old patient starved himself to death over a 47-day period. But who would seriously want to suggest that it is in the patient's best interests to be dehydrated and starved to death? It appears that the World Medical Assembly and the American President's Commission would.[15]

If there is no moral difference in favor of passive euthanasia (causing death by nonintervention), over active euthanasia (causing death by intervention) it is illogical to accept the former and reject the latter; and if there is, as has been suggested, a moral difference in favor of active euthanasia, the consensus of medical opinion is immoral as well.

In the case of the competent patient who, in addition to an interest in general well-being, also has an interest in self-determination, the inconsistency of the Commission's position is even more glaringly obvious, since it treats a competent person's interest in and right to self-determination as paramount. Competent patients should be allowed to die, it says, when from their point of view, life in a distressing or seriously debilitating condition is no longer worthwhile. Different people will decide differently when this point has been reached. Since normal adult persons have an *overriding* interest in the exercise of their "capacity to form, revise and pursue his or her own plans for life," "no uniform, objective determination can be adequate whether defined by society or by health care professionals."[16] But there is no suggestion that the competent person whose right to self-determination is paramount is to be allowed to die at a time and in a manner of his or her own choosing if this requires, as it often does, the cooperation of others.

Postscript

I have been arguing that changes in the law of Common Law jurisdictions are urgent and that such changes are unlikely to be brought about unless they have the support of the medical profession, the majority of which holds to an illogical acceptance of passive, and rejection of active euthanasia. To judge from opinion polls, public opinion is very much more liberal on these issues; but opinion polls are notoriously unreliable since the respondents are often unaware of the complexities of the issues underlying the questions put. Other evidence suggests that the general public is, on the whole, indifferent. For example, the membership of the 27 "Right to Die" societies that exist in 17 countries remains very small, though it is growing fast.

What we need to bring about is a change in our whole society's attitude towards death and dying. Instead of sweeping it under the carpet (many North Americans who are in other respects not mealy-mouthed use euphemisms for "death"), we must relearn to accept death, as our forefathers did, as not only the inevitable, but the natural end to earthly life. My ideal death is that of Socrates who took poison and died discussing the immortality of the soul with his friends. To be sure, his reason for choosing to die was that he had been condemned to death by the laws of his country which he felt bound to obey. But change that story a little. Socrates is growing old; he can no longer handle his stonemason's tools with the old skill; worse still, he can no longer match his friends in philosophic discussion. Life has no more that he values to offer him; so he accepts death, not knowing what is to come, having enjoyed life to the end.

NOTES

1. British Medical Association, *Handbook of Medical Ethics* (1980), 31.
2. John Dawson, "An Open and Gentle Death," British Medical Association, *News Review*, vol. 12, no. 1, January 1986, 22.
3. Pieter V. Admiraal, "Active Voluntary Euthanasia," The Voluntary Euthanasia Society, *Newsletter*, no. 24 (London, May 1985).
4. Dawson, *op. cit.*, 23.
5. Law Reform Commission of Canada, *Euthanasia, Suicide and Cessation Treatment* (Ottawa, 1984) (Emphasis added).
6. *Ibid.*
7. The Voluntary Euthanasia Society, *Newsletter* no. 24 (London, May 1985), 5.
8. *Ibid.*, no. 23, 1–2.
9. *The Sunday Times* (London, 16 December 1984).
10. Aristotle, *Nicomachean Ethics*, III, 1110a.
11. Statement of terminal illness and boxing, October 1983. *Medical Journal of Australia*, 1984, vol. 141, 549. I am indebted for this and the following references to Dr. Helga Kuhse of the Center for Human Bioethics, Monash University, Australia.
12. "Deciding to Forego Life-Sustaining Treatment" (Washington, U.S. Government Printing Office, 1983).
13. Helga Kuhse, "Euthanasia—Again," *Medical Journal of Australia*, 1985, vol. 142, 612.
14. Quoted by Peter Singer and Helga Kuhse, "The Future of Baby Doe," *New York Review of Books*, 1984, 31, 17–22.
15. Helga Kuhse, *op.cit.*, 611.
16. *Ibid.*, 612.

JUSTIFIED WARFARE and the RELATIVE VALUE Of HUMAN LIFE

Peter van den Dungen

Warfare, like some other social institutions and practices which have a direct bearing on human life, has a long history—in fact, the oldest history we have is that which records the waging of war, which is not surprising since "history began as tales of martial exploits written down by court chroniclers to immortalize the glory of their master."[1] Reflection on the ethical dimensions of this particular practice, including speculation on the justification for the sacrifice of human life thus exacted, has a less extended history which starts at the latest with the emergence of the great religions in East and West and which promulgated general rules affecting various social practices and behavior, including war. In the Western world, we can consider as milestones in the debate on this subject the teachings of the Church Fathers (especially St. Augustine) and of Thomas Aquinas; the further development of the theory of the Just War by 16th-century Spanish theologians (culminating in the 1625 treatise on international law by

Grotius); the social doctrines and practices of certain churches which emerged in the Reformation period and afterwards (such as Anabaptists or Mennonites and Quakers); and the Christian-based peace movement which arose in the aftermath of the Napoleonic wars in America and England.

A considerable body of literature on the ethics of war thus exists; it can broadly be summarized in two distinct schools of thought: a qualified acceptance of war (the "just war" doctrine) traditionally has prevailed over an absolute rejection of it ("pacifism"). Changes in the nature of modern weapons and warfare, particularly since 1945, have brought about a marked shift in the relative acceptance of both points of view. In fact, a new division has arisen within the larger framework of a general rejection of war (at any rate between the main powers) and in which the retention of the tools of war (in their most developed form) has become the issue. While there is widespread agreement that nuclear war is indefensible (and that conventional war may escalate into nuclear war), there is great argument concerning the best means to prevent the outbreak of war, revolving around the moral acceptability of nuclear deterrence. The paradox contained in the traditional maxim, *Si vis pacem, para bellum,* has assumed an almost unbearable poignancy because of the nature of the preparation for war and the price—not the least in moral terms—which is likely to be paid in the event of deterrence failing.

On such vital questions as that of the value, preservation and integrity of human life, it is tempting to look for, and expect to find, consistency in the attitude which an individual person or social group (be it a political party, religious organization, or even an entire culture), holds on such diverse life-and-death matters as infanticide, capital punishment, euthanasia, dueling and war. However, consistency is often lacking, allowing, for instance, a critic of current peace movement to write to its members: "Their ethical eclecticism, indeed opportunism, entangles them sometimes in contradictions: some Green Peace fighters, for instance, praise life as the highest good and at the same time defend abortion,"[2] or a leading British antinuclear campaigner, Monsignor Bruce Kent, to write of his church that he "cannot see why a church that holds views of such certainty and clarity on issues like abortion is not just as unequivocal about the sin inherent in the ownership of weapons capable of destroying the world."[3] Equally, one could refer to the "Moral Right" today whose "prolife" agenda includes both a condemnation of abortion and a strong commitment to deterrence, including willingness to go to war—and hence to kill not one potential life but potentially all life. A curious case of inconsistency in ethical reasoning and behavior which has arisen in recent years is presented by the extreme wing of the animal rights movement which has, quite literally, declared war on vivisection. In Britain, the Animal Liberation Front, with its hard, terrorist edge, believes that direct action, involving not only the destruction of property but even of human life, is morally justified in a war to free the animals which are now being used and abused for reasons of food, sport and medical research.[4]

Such inconsistencies, however, glaring as they may be, are not new and can be found throughout history—what changes are the concrete issues and causes but not the anomaly or inconsistency in the thinking about them. Just as in previous eras, those who condemned slavery, the death penalty, or the duel, but not war, were invited to reconsider their acceptance of this practice (and vice versa: there were those who condemned war but not some of the other practices which involved the taking of life), so today attitudes on war are often juxtaposed to those on abortion or euthanasia—as an argument to persuade others of the error of their ways. The uneven, erratic development of the moral sensibilities of individuals, societies and entire civilizations or epochs and the way this reflected in their social customs and institutions can, in a general sense, be regarded as an illustration of Mannheim's notion of the "contemporaneity of the noncontemporaneous,"[5] which is a characteristic of probably all societies, not only in the moral but also, e.g., in the intellectual and material fields.

In his *History of European Morals*, the great Irish historian Lecky has observed:

> There are in human nature, and more especially in the exercise of the benevolent affections, inequalities, inconsistencies and anomalies.... We have a much greater power than is sometimes supposed of localizing both our benevolent and malevolent feelings.... Our affections are so capricious in their nature that it is continually necessary to correct by detailed experience the most plausible deductions.[6]

He relates how, during the Roman Empire with its gladiatorial combats, "The very men who looked down with delight when the sand of the arena was reddened with human blood, made the theater ring with applause when Terence, in his famous line, proclaimed the universal brotherhood of man."[7] Another popular spectacle in ancient Rome was ropedancing, high above the ground. When, in the reign of Marcus Aurelius, an accident occurred, the emperor ordered that henceforth no ropedancer should perform without a net or a mattress being spread out below. "It is a singularly curious fact," Lecky writes, "that this precaution, which no Christian nation has adopted, continued in force during more than a century of the worst period of the Roman Empire, when the blood of captives was poured out like water in the Colosseum."[8] The difficulty of making "plausible deductions" regarding an individual's attitude to life, Lecky also abundantly illustrates with respect to what is now called "speciescism." Animal liberationists would not have approved of Spinoza, "one of the purest, most gentle, most benevolent of mankind, of whom it is related that almost the only amusement of his life was putting flies into spiders' webs, and watching their struggles and their deaths."[9] On the other hand, "It has been observed that a very large proportion of the men who during the French Revolution proved themselves most absolutely indifferent to human suffering were deeply attached to animals."[10]

We may stay with Lecky for another moment and report his views on the impact of Christianity on the question of the sanctity of human life. He writes:

> The first aspect in which Christianity presented itself to the world was as a declaration of the fraternity of men in Christ...the first and most manifest duty of a Christian man was to look upon his fellowmen as sacred beings, and from this notion grew the eminently Christian idea of the sanctity of all human life.[11]

Lecky emphasizes the novelty of this notion since

> nature does not tell man that it is wrong to slay without provocation his fellowmen...it is an historical fact beyond all dispute that refined, and even moral, societies have existed in which the slaughter of men of some particular class or nation has been regarded with no more compunction that the slaughter of animals in the chase.[12]

Christianity set a new standard, higher than any which then existed in the world, and its influence affected a whole range of social practices, starting with the very earliest stage of human life and including, at the other end of the spectrum, war. Christians denounced abortion in the strongest terms "not simply as inhuman, but as definitely murder."[13] Lecky similarly documents the beneficent influence of the new religion on infanticide, slavery, war,[14] gladiatorial shows and suicide. As regards the latter, virgins were permitted to commit suicide in order to avoid rape, although Augustine disapproved of this exception and with him the doctrine of the absolute sinfulness of suicide became generally accepted by Catholic theologians. But as Lecky points out, "by a glaring though very natural inconsistency, no characters were more enthusiastically extolled than those anchorites who habitually deprived their bodies of the sustenance that was absolutely necessary to health, and thus manifestly abridged their lives."[15] The doctrine of the sanctity of human life seemed to be infringed not only by these "slow suicides" but also by the self-torture which was a distinguishing characteristic of the "ascetic epidemic" which affected Christianity in the fourth and fifth centuries.[16]

A history of moral thought and practice reveals, as the above has briefly sought to indicate, the presence of paradoxes and anomalies. We may now go on to address more specifically the question of war—the moral issues involved in its traditional practice and, conversely, in that of its complete renunciation. Some episodes from the history of pacifism—the doctrine which, in its extreme form, proclaims the absolute inviolability of human life—will serve as a starting point. The implications of such a doctrine, the difficulties inherent in its consistent application, and the arguments which have been put forward in opposition to it, will be briefly reviewed. The movement for the abolition of war was, for a considerable time, functioning in a society which fully accepted the institution of slavery. Even within Quakerism, this inconsistency persisted for a long time. Peter Brock has commented that "an awareness of inconsistency between Friends' principles and the practice of slave-holding only ripened slowly."[17] John Woolman (1720–1772) was one of those most responsible for launching the Society of Friends on its antislavery path. He drew attention to "the implicit hypocrisy of asserting the wrongfulness of all wars and at the same time holding in bondage fellowmen whose subjection was the result of armed force."[18] The French-born Quaker Anthony Benezet similarly asked in 1754 of his fellow Quakers, "How can we, who have been concerned to publish the gospel of universal love and peace among mankind, be so inconsistent with ourselves as to purchase such who are prisoners of war...?"[19] Thomas Grimké, who was a leading figure in the absolutist wing of the American Peace Society (to the extent of even regarding the American Revolution as being "utterly indefensible"), was, at the time of his death in 1834, still an owner of slaves (although Brock writes that he was just beginning to give the whole question of slavery his serious consideration and that, had he lived, he would have become an abolitionist like his two sisters).[20]

Among advocates of the abolition of war, the demand for consistency, exemplified in the above, was, however, far from universally shared. It is perhaps not an exaggeration to say that a striking feature from the history of the opposition to war was the failure of the attempt to attach to war a unique moral stigma and, thus, to isolate it from other social customs and institutions which were considered wrong and evil. Such attempts were made in the organized peace movement of the 19th century in order to attract as many supporters as possible. If adherence to the causes of the elimination of slavery and of the death penalty also was to be implied in the movement to abolish war, the latter might not have attracted many sympathizers at a time when all three institutions were widespread and taken for granted—but when peace societies considered war to be the greatest abomination.[21] George C. Beckwith, the long-serving secretary of the American Peace Society in the middle decades of the 19th century, expressed this view very clearly in his introduction to Thomas Upham's *The Manual of Peace*, the first edition of which was published 150 years ago in 1836:

> We wish the cause of Peace to be distinctly understood. It seeks only the abolition of a specific, well-defined custom—the practice of international war—has nothing to do with anything else.... This view of our cause relieves it from a variety of extraneous questions.... We (have) nothing to do with capital punishments, or the strict inviolability of human life, or the question whether the gospel allows the application

of physical force to the government of states, schools and families. We go merely against war; and war is defined by our best lexicographers to be "a contest by force between nations."[22]

Upham himself, however, writing within the rigid framework of the fundamentalist, literalist interpretation of the Bible, frequently referred in his book to the prohibition contained in the Sixth Commandment. God, he says, "has made use of the most general terms, clearly asserting the inviolability of human life in all cases whatever."[23] "The doctrine of the absolute inviolability of human life," he writes, "is not yet victorious but will soon be."[24]

Some 10 years later, Beckwith wrote his own *The Peace Manual*, partly "to counteract some dangerous notions to be found in the earlier *Manual of Peace*."[25] These dangerous notions concerned the views of absolute pacifists and nonresistants who denied not only the inadmissibility of defensive war (as Beckwith did), but also the right of governments to coerce in internal politics. These issues had deeply divided the American Peace Society in the previous years; under Beckwith's leadership the moderates established their authority. The essence of their argument is stated in Beckwith's preface to his own volume and which is very similar to the one he had contributed to Upham's *Manual*:

> The cause of peace aims solely to do away the custom of international war; and I trust there will be found in this book nothing that does not bear on this object, nor anything that interferes with the legitimate authority of government. As a friend of peace, I am of course a supporter of civil government. As a friend of peace, I am of course a supporter of civil government, with all the powers requisite for the condign punishment of wrongdoers, the enforcement of law, and the preservation of social order.[26]

The condemnation of defensive war (the most contentious issue between the moderates and radicals in the American Peace Society) by many Christian pacifists was based on an extension to international life of the teaching that it was morally wrong for Christians to quarrel and fight, instead of returning good for evil. That there were wars of aggression and wars of defense (or "just" wars) they regarded as a delusion and a specious argument: all wars were wars of aggression. To the question what was to happen when a nation was under foreign attack, their answer was: (a) obey God's command, i.e., resist from doing evil; (b) trust in His protection; (c) be ready to suffer martyrdom. Some, such as Grimké, made the familiar point that any justification of defensive war by drawing an analogy with the function of the magistrate in a nation's domestic affairs was misleading since no supranational community and no international code of law was in existence.[27] Nations would be judge, jury and executioner in their own cause. With the growth of international law and organization, some pacifists have conceded the decreasing validity of Grimké's argument and have gone on to sanction the use of force in the hands of a legitimate "international magistrate." Brock correctly identifies one of the main reasons for the unconvincing nature of the rejection by most 19th-century pacifists of defensive war. Beckwith, like many peace advocates of his day, "was reasoning on the assumption that all wars (between civilized nations, at least) were, with a little patience and goodwill, avoidable...the deeper implications raised by wars of national liberation or by ideological conflict or the will toward aggression...were...ignored."[28]

Beckwith's decided assertion of the inadmissibility of any war, combined with his equally firm rejection (in public, if not in private) of the principle of the inviolability of human life in domestic affairs, invited criticisms from both the conservative and the radical wings of the Society over which he presided. He regarded civil government as "lawful, expedient and necessary" and in no way incompatible with the renunciation of force between nations. Civil government had been ordained by God, and as the instrument of his justice it must be endowed with the means of enforcing its will upon the refractory—and for this it was permissible to inflict even death itself. But if Beckwith could countenance the punishment, with death even, by the government of a Christian country of a score of pirates or of half a dozen murderers, and the suppression with armed force of an insurrection, why, conservative and moderate opponents asked, could it be wrong for such a government to repel by arms an invading army intent upon robbing and killing? His answer lacked conviction:

> God permits the taking of life in one case, but not in the other. He
> authorizes rulers to govern, but not to fight; to punish, but not to

quarrel. Such acts, even if they were physically the same, would be morally different; and, hence, one *may* be permitted, while the other is forbidden.[29]

Moreover, whereas civil government aimed at establishing justice among men, the outcome of war was quite different, since war was "no more than a rencounter [sic] between tigers."[30]

Critics of Beckwith's position argued that it was inconsistent: for a Christian, either life was held to be inviolable, in which case the use of coercive force by a government stood also condemned and nonresistance was the only possible attitude, or it was not, and in that case both domestic force and defensive war were permitted. The arbitrary nature of the division between external and internal affairs which Beckwith had tried to argue was pointedly exposed by the Rev. John Lord who asked, in 1839,

> When does protection begin and end, and how many men does it take to make a mob, and where is the difference on the grand principle, between a foreign and domestic body of robbers and murderers? Do we not enforce the same principle in regard to a multitude of foreign enemies that we do of domestic ones?.... The doctrine that *all* war is opposed to the gospel *does* run into nonresistance. It is vain and trifling to deny it.[31]

Twenty years earlier, John Sheppard had made the same point by focusing on the difficulty caused by the word "war." His eloquent words may be quoted at some length since they go to the heart of the matter:

> The truth is, unless it be proved that every war has been unjust and criminal on both sides, *war* is a name adapted to produce confusion of idea; because it includes *contrary things*, aggression and defense, crime and punishment. I grant the fact to be that *most* wars *have* been unjust on both sides, which has led to this indiscriminate name, and that they have generally deserved to be stigmatized with a confounding appellation.... But still, while it is certain that there have been, and may be, wars in which the crime is as clearly on one side as in a riot or robbery, it is as unfit that the name *war* should be applied to both parties, as the name *riot*, or *robbery*, to the forcible acts of the *civil power*, which restrains or suppresses them. We cannot, however, change the language of mankind; but it is sophistical to avail ourselves of its ambiguity.[32]

A few words must be devoted to those who criticized Beckwith's position from an absolutist stance since interesting lessons can be drawn from their fate. The great abolitionist (of slavery, to be sure), William Lloyd Garrison (1805–1879), was the spokesman of those who came to believe that the logical outcome of Christian pacifism was a renunciation of all association with the state; the doctrine of nonresistance implied a renunciation of civil government altogether and the adoption of political anarchism. Garrison and his followers split from the American Peace Society in 1838 and formed the New England Non-Resistance Society, which resolved "that human life is inviolable, and can never be taken by individuals or nations without committing sin against God." Not only the armed forces and the police, but the whole apparatus of government, was rejected as being incompatible with Christianity. When Civil War came, Garrison proved unable, however, to combine truthfully his advocacy of abolition with the maintenance of pacifism and nonresistance. His paper, *The Liberator*, vigorously supported persecution of the war and opposed concessions to the South; the bellicosity and irreconcilable tone of the paper contrasted strangely with Garrison's theoretical pacifism and his insistence that he was in no way compromising his peace principles. He failed to see any incompatibility between theory and practice in his conduct, telling a friend who deplored what he regarded as Garrison's lapse from the spirit, if not the letter, of nonviolence: "Although nonresistance holds human life in all cases inviolable, yet it is perfectly consistent for those professing it to petition, advise, and strenuously urge a pro-war government to abolish slavery solely by the war-power."[33]

The Grimké sisters, prominent Quakers, abolitionists and one-time nonresisters provide another illustration (among many others) of how the most fervent apostles of nonviolence turned into the most rabid enthusiasts of slave revolt and civil war. "You see how warlike I have become.... Oh, yes—war is better than slavery," wrote Angelina in 1862; and in a letter to Garrison in 1864, her sister Sarah spoke of "This blessed war.... This war, the holiest ever waged, is emphatically God's war."[34] Their experience demonstrates the validity of Ralph Potter's observation that those who reject the just war theory in favor of an absolute pacifism are in danger of falling victim to the crusading mentality when they abandon their pacifism. Having never been accustomed to thinking in terms of the discriminating categories of just war, the *jus in bello* is unlikely to restrain those now zealous in a worthy cause. "Those who adhere to the ethic of the saint must never, never indulge in war," he cautions, "for they will then have no habitual modes of moral discrimination to guard them from committing barbarities under the guise of their presumed virtuous intent."[35] Yet, in Potter's felicitous phrase, "Force must always be restrained because its only legitimate function is to restrain."[36] He is right in stressing that the just war doctrine, which is the precipitate of moral reflection upon political experience in the West, is valid whenever violence is at issue, and provides an ethic for the policeman and the magistrate, as well as the soldier.[37] Through compromise, the just war theory acknowledges what is best in the extreme attitudes of pacifism (the concern for life) and crusades (the protection of the innocent, of justice, etc.). Reinhold Niebuhr similarly has pointed out the dangers of moral absolutism in politics, arguing that "The political order must be satisfied with relative peace and relative justice."[38]

If the Civil War had managed to turn ultrapacifists into warmongers, it is not surprising to find the American Peace Society (which aimed to be a "broad church") rallied to the support of the Northern war effort as soon as fighting began. The argument of the pro-war majority was simply that the conflict, which had broken out between the government and the Southern states, did not come under the heading of war and that, therefore, it did not come under the ban of the Society. It was a rebellion and the suppression of rebellion was a legitimate task of government and should have the full backing of the Society. If the use of armed force to put down the rebels was contrary to Christianity, the *Advocate of Peace* (the Society's organ) wrote in 1861, "then all real, effective government is wrong, and society must be abandoned to a remediless, everlasting anarchy."[39] As Peter Brock has commented, the Society's reasoning—war is war between nations, civil war is not war but police action—was sophistical. In truth, war fever had swamped the American Peace Society, and only a handful of stalwarts opposed the war as being un-Christian and incompatible with the aims and teachings of the Society.[40]

The travails of the American Peace Society (and of the remnants of the New England Non-Resistance Society, its radical offshoot) during the American Civil War provide one illustration among many of the correctness of John Lewis's argument that "Pacifism flourishes behind the lines, far from the battlefront.... Very many pacifists, perhaps most, would lose their pacifism in an instant if anything they seriously valued were threatened by violence."[41] Many of Lewis's contemporaries were quick to prove his point since they abandoned their pacifism when faced with the Nazi threat. Then they suddenly shared his opinion that circumstances "may make some wars better than peace...A bad peace may be worse than a good war"[42]—even though, until recently, they had firmly endorsed Benjamin Franklin's opinion that "there never was a good war, or a bad peace" (a sentiment already expressed by Cicero—"I cease not to advocate peace: even though unjust it is better than the justest war").[43] They rejected a peace which, while avoiding war, was likely to result in the loss of liberty and the imposition of slavery. As John Oman wrote in the 1930s:

> To treat a man as a chattel is a much graver denial that he is an end in himself than to say to him: You must die, as I should be willing to die in like case, rather than live as the instrument for giving victory to an unrighteous cause. To enslave others is always an acuter opposition to the whole Christian order than fighting others, unless we are merely fighting to enslave them. To make life an end in itself and to make a man an end in himself are things so different that every good by which a man's soul is saved must be valued above life; and freedom, the condition of truly possessing a soul, no man can ever have except by setting it above life.[44]

The fact that many, perhaps most, wars have been waged in causes which cannot be regarded as just, and that much blood had been spilt lightly and immorally, does not diminish the truth and enduring appeal of this insight. Equally, when the British Conservative Chancellor of the Exchequer, Sir Michael Hicks Beach, in a speech during the Fashoda Crisis (1898), said that if the outcome would be war it would be a great calamity—"But there are greater evils than war" (thereby, apparently, popularizing this maxim)—the truth contained in it is a matter altogether separate from its application.[45] The relative fortunes of England and France in their bids for imperialistic hegemony in Africa at the turn of the century was definitely not a matter which would have justified the recourse to war.

It is not only the threat of an impending evil which can bring about the sudden conversion which Lewis has noticed; the promise of removing an *existing* evil can have the same effect, as we have seen demonstrated above in the American Civil War. In such concrete circumstances, the difficulties inherent in maintaining an absolute pacifism (one which judges the wrongfulness of war not by consequences but by eternal and absolute principles, or which proclaims that war is always evil and that good can never come out of evil) become evident, as does the ambiguous nature of "war." Echoing John Sheppard, Lewis writes: "War, like every other evil, is not just of one kind...a war [is] good or bad according to its purpose and result. It is, therefore, a complete fallacy to characterize *war* as either good or bad in itself."[46] In rejecting absolute pacifism and arguing instead for a utilitarian pacifism, Lewis takes as his supreme law, not the inviolability of human life, but the principle of love, the desire that we shall do men good rather than harm. This, he says,

> may involve us in the taking of human life. We cannot, therefore, say that violence in itself, or killing in itself, is invariably morally wrong, though it is, of course, always evil.... War is an evil, as all admit, but it is right if the evil it avoids is a greater evil, and that has to be determined in each particular case.[47]

He argues that "violence, while it always remains evil, is not a moral wrong, but a moral duty, where it results in a balance of human welfare, as for instance where it is used to protect an innocent victim, to restrain anarchy and violence, or to maintain a just social order."[48] The *moral* character of a violent act has to be distinguished from its purely physical character: while the latter remains the same, the former depends on motive and purpose.[49] It is this distinction which allows another one, commonly denied by pacifists, namely that between killing murder. That in war, "killing is not murder" presupposes that both the resort to war and the manner of its conduct are in strict accordance with the principles of the just war theory.

Augustine, writing that "there are some exceptions made by the divine authority to its own law, that men may not be put to death," taught that persons who wage war at God's command (sic) or who slay evil men in their capacity as public officials "have by no means violated the commandment 'Thou shalt not kill.'"[50] He justifies the existence of coercive powers ("the power of the king, the right of life and death exercised by the judge, the hooks of the executioner, the weapons of the soldier") as a means whereby "evil men are held in check, and the good live more peacefully among the wicked."[51] For Augustine, as for Thomas Aquinas nine centuries later, the object of war was peace. In this context, it is also relevant to refer to Augustine's view that the real evil in war is not death but "the love of violence, revengeful cruelty, fierce and implacable enmity, wild resistance and the lust of power, and such like." These are the things (rather than death) which makes war evil because they bring death to the soul, not merely to the body. The fact that Augustine insisted on the principle that physical death is neither the end of life nor the greatest evil, and that he regarded war and the suffering of the innocent as inevitable, does not mean that he displayed a lack of concern over the death of innocent people in war.[52]

The belief that "killing is not murder" is not uniquely applied to the institution of warfare but also underlies other social practices which involve the deliberate taking of human life. Apart from the fact that such practices are (or have been) legally sanctioned, what are some of the social and psychological factors which account for the easiness with which individuals accept and act upon this belief in warfare? The abrogation of the normal taboo on killing fellow human beings (and its replacement by a duty to kill them), is psychologically symbolized by the wearing of uniforms. Even in our age of sophisticated, technological warfare, the warrior's traditional war paint and plumes survive in unobtrusive forms such as stars, chevrons and buttons. Arnold Toynbee has commented that this dressing up for war look childish but that its continued survival reveals two important functions: the psychological one, already referred to, and the practical one of enabling a visual distinction between the soldier and the civilian (although the growth of total warfare has made the latter distinction increasingly difficult and irrelevant). "The moral sense of mankind in general has been obtuse enough to regard the killer in war as being righteous—at least, so long as he keeps, more or less faithfully, to the recognized rules," writes Toynbee.[53] He rightly refrains from making too categorical a statement as there are exceptions to the general rule, he notes. Freud has pointed out, e.g., that the prohibition to kill, the result of mankind's awakening conscience, was gradually extended outwards and ultimately came to include unloved strangers and even enemies. Although this final extension is no longer experienced by civilized man, it is

> worthy of note that such primitive races as still inhabit the earth act differently in this respect; when (the savage) returns victorious from the warpath he may not set foot in his village nor touch his wife until he has atoned for the murders committed in war by penances which are often prolonged and toilsome. This may be presumed, of course, to be the outcome of superstition.[54]

But behind this, Freud contends, "lurks a vein of ethical sensitiveness which has been lost by us civilized men."

In "Our Attitude towards Death," which forms the second part of the essay we have quoted from, Freud discusses the changes which war causes in the participant's attitude, not only as regards the taking of life but also the giving up of his own life. Since war inevitably involves both phenomena, an enquiry concerning the relative value of human life in warfare cannot avoid considering the individual's motives for sacrificing his own life (as distinct from taking his opponent's). We shall confine ourselves to some observations which have commonly been made in this respect and which stress deepseated psychological reasons (rather than the obvious and publicly-claimed ones, such as the preservation or achievement of such fundamental values as justice, liberty, freedom and—less prominent today—honor and glory for oneself or one's country). Freud argues that death has been exorcised from normal life in the West, appearing as an accident rather than as an unavoidable necessity, and that this taboo has a powerful effect upon our lives:

> Life is impoverished, it loses in interest, when the highest stake in the game of living, life itself, may not be risked.... The tendency to exclude

death from our calculations brings in its train a number of other renunciations and exclusions. And yet the motto of the Hanseatic League declared: *"Navigare necesse est, vivere non necesse!"* (It is necessary to sail the seas, it is not necessary to live.)[55]

War, however, sweeps away this conventional attitude to death: it can no longer be denied and "life has, in truth, become interesting again; it has regained its full significance."[56]

That war seems to offer an outlet for drives and emotions which are normally suppressed is confirmed by other psychologists, notably William James, who believes that we will only be successful in our attempts to eliminate war if we are aware of the basic functions which war apparently fulfills and if we can find a "moral equivalent" for it. War enables those involved to experience feelings of community and comradeship which are seldom attained in normal life and for which, nevertheless, there is a deep longing. It seems that such feelings only can be attained as a result of some extreme experience, usually involving mortal danger. The American philosopher J. Glenn Gray, who has reflected on his own war experience, writes: "How does danger break down the barriers of the self and give man an experience of community? The answer to this question is the key to one of the oldest and most enduring incitements to battle."[57] With James, he believes that "there are surely alternative ways more creative and less dreadful, if men would only seek them out."[58] (Later on, however, he is not so sure: "The ways of peace have not found—perhaps cannot find—substitutes for the communal enthusiasm and ecstasies of war.")[59] Gray makes a distinction between external reasons from fighting, such reasons being to fight and die for one's country, or religion, or any other abstract good, and the concrete circumstances of battle which involve the decision to be killed. Here he observes that "Numberless soldiers have died, more or less willingly...because they realized that by fleeing their post and rescuing themselves, they would expose their companions to greater danger."[60] When Hannah Arendt writes in her introduction to Gray's book that the soldier's basic credo is "that life is *not* the highest good,"[61] this does not always imply more than that he is sacrificing his life for the physical survival of his comrade. Gray adds that "the assurance of immortality...makes self-sacrifice at these moments so relatively easy."[62]

Self-sacrifice is found in war as in other spheres of life, in the first place the religious one. The similarities between war and religion have frequently been commented on: just as war has been regarded as a religious activity—surrounded as it is by prayer, ritual, sacrifice and purification[63]—and defended in terms of devotion and salvation, so religion has often adopted a military terminology and character.[64] The true believer, whether he be a soldier (assuming that he has fully accepted the "external" reasons for war) or a saint or martyr, must be ready to give up his life for the faith. "And if he is a genuine saint, he will regard this sacrifice as no loss, for the self has become indestructible in being united with a supreme reality."[65] This, Gray continues, "is the mystical element that has been mentioned by nearly all serious writers on the subject;" it is the boundless capacity for self-sacrifice that is intoxicating about war.

Apart from what constitutes the "enduring appeal of battle" (which, in Gray's analysis, includes next to comradeship, love of the spectacle and of destruction), Gray's reflections also touch on images of "the enemy"—the abstractness of the term permitting the growth of abstract hatred. One of the many paradoxes of war is that the further a person is from dangerous contact with this image, the more he is consumed by it. Several common attitudes toward the enemy can be distinguished in wars of recent times; those in which the enemy is regarded as a creature which is not human but a species of animal pest, or that which depicts the enemy as the devil or devil possessed, obviously reduce any inhibitions about killing him. In fact, such killing may be profoundly satisfying, since war assumes the character of a mission, a holy cause.[66] A different factor which enables killing is the drugged state so common in combat, the result of training and fatigue, which makes soldiers act as automatons.[67] Denis Winter, describing the experiences of soldiers in World War I, also frequently refers to the "self-drugged state" in which they advanced and fought, and which was partly caused by the upset in body chemistry produced by a state of high fear long sustained.[68] He quotes one soldier who observed, "God is merciful and it almost seems as though he chloroforms us on these occasions;" another one felt he had gone through the battle "like a sleepwalker."

Winter adds: "There are incidents recalled beyond number in memoirs in which men wondered if it was really themselves who gouged, clawed, clubbed and bayoneted. How could they have behaved so wildly?"[69]

Some of the above observations by Freud and Gray lose their meaning and import when the context is "nuclear death." This possibility has reduced to absurd cliches the fine words of the past when men proposed to die with honor rather than to live in shame because there would be nobody left to honor the dead. A defense of freedom and civilization at the price of destroying them is similarly absurd. In his essay "Death in the Nuclear Age," Morgenthau has written that it is "this contrast between our consciousness and the objective conditions in which we live, the backwardness of our consciousness in view of the possibility of nuclear death, that threatens us with the actuality of nuclear death."[70] This is the unique predicament of our age which faces the double challenge of totalitarian encroachment and nuclear devastation. Richard Falk has perceptively noted that "The risks of the age burden us with the moral necessity to meet both challenges, although meeting one too ardently leads to an increased vulnerability to the other."[71] Indeed, this challenge cannot be resolved by believing that there is an easy way out of this dilemma, or by asking "whether war is a greater or lesser evil than the imposition...of hostile values which the present anarchic world, with its attendant threat of war, allows...to keep at a distance."[72] Assuming the impossibility of a meaningful victory and survival following a major nuclear war, such a war is a greater evil than any conceivable alternative since it would destroy mankind and civilization.[73]

F.S. Northedge is confusing the issue when he writes that it is not clear whether Bertrand Russell "really wishes to pay the price of global despotism in return for peace" since "elsewhere, he writes that a new war would be preferable to a universal communist empire."[74] Russell's case is an exceedingly interesting one which, as in this quote, has often been misunderstood. In "The Future of Mankind," an essay written shortly after the end of World War II and of the failure of the Baruch plan, Russell suggested that the U.S. use the threat of force and, if need be, actual force, in order to bring about a world government as the only means to monopolize atomic power and thus prevent the end of civilization in a future atomic world war. In this bold, timely and farsighted essay, he wrote that

> beyond the difficulties and probable tragedies of the near future there is the possibility of immeasurable good, and of greater well-being than has ever before fallen to the lot of man. This is not merely a possibility, but, if the Western democracies are firm and prompt, a probability.[75]

This suggestion was not acted upon and when, in 1949, the Soviet Union exploded a nuclear device, the genie was out of the bottle, and Russell's idea had become obsolete. In the late 1950s, Russell became a prominent figure in the British nuclear disarmament campaign and was accused by some of inconsistency. But as he wrote, "My critics seem to think that, if you have once advocated a certain policy, you should continue to advocate it after all the circumstances have changed. This is quite absurd."[76] In an age of nuclear proliferation, in which nuclear war spells suicide, the most elementary freedom is the freedom to choose survival, he wrote, criticizing those who argued that "No World" was preferable to a communist or a capitalist world. Those who held the latter opinion, he advised to question their right "to impose their opinion upon those who do not hold it by the infliction of the death penalty upon all of them." This was, he concluded, an extreme form of religious persecution, never witnessed in human history.[77]

What Russell advocated briefly at one time could be regarded as "aggressive" war and one, moreover, in which the Americans were presumably entitled, if need be, to use the atomic weapon. Even such a war Russell would have regarded as "justified" in order to avoid later a much greater catastrophe which he thought very likely.[78] It is pertinent to point out that in this respect (the possible justification of offensive war), Russell shared the views of his main opponent[79] in the celebrated exchange on the morality of war which took place largely in the pages of the *International Journal of Ethics* during 1915. Russell initiated this debate with his article "The Ethics of War," in which he justified his "pacifist" stand and argued that none of the combatants in the war then taking place had a just cause. He admitted that war was not always a crime: what was important and decisive was not whether treaties had been broken and whether, on paper, a war was justified but whether there was a real justification for it "in the balance of good which it is to bring to mankind." This was the only valid criterion, and applying it to the past, he found that wars had taken place in which the good of mankind outweighed all the evils of war; the present war was not among them.[80] Ralph Barton Perry, professor of philosophy at Harvard, criticized Russell's nonresistance for being incompatible with his desire to preserve what is valuable in national life. Perry argued that "to try out this principle of nonresistance one must imagine the greatest conceivable good to be attacked with a deliberate intent to destroy it; or the greatest conceivable evil to be threatened with a deliberate and implacable intent to perpetrate it."[81] To believe, as Russell did, that all things British—its civilization, democracy, language, and manufacture—could survive defeat and occupation was unrealistic. Later, Russell was implicitly to concede this when he wrote, "When, in 1940, England was threatened with invasion, I realized that, throughout the First War, I had never seriously envisaged the possibility of utter defeat. I found this possibility unbearable, and at last consciously definitely decided that I must support what was necessary for victory in the Second War."[82] He had, he now recognized, allowed a larger sphere to the method of nonresistance than later experience (also in his personal life) seemed to warrant. Still, he could rightly claim that "the practical difference, between [my] opposing the First War and supporting the Second, was so great as to mask the considerable degree of theoretical consistency that in fact existed."[83] The difference between Perry and Russell was, likewise, not one of principle but of its application. They both hated war, and to Perry's claim that "the cause for which one may properly make war is the cause of peace," Russell replied, in agreement, "that it is legitimate to make war in order to end war."[84]

The initial enthusiasm for the Great War on the part of the peoples in the Allied countries was the belief that, in the words of H.G. Wells, this "is not just another war—it is the last war."[85] The title of his book, *The War that will End War,* is symptomatic of the inflated moral idealism with which the British, and later the Americans, justified their participation in the war. In a stimulating (but not always very balanced) essay on "War and The

242

Philosopher's Duty," Warren Steinkraus has argued that one duty of the philosopher is precisely to clear up the confusing and misleading language of politics and of value which surrounds war.[86] The unending talk of freedom in World War II contrasts sharply, he writes, with the practice of the "free world" which, as in the case of Britain, maintained a colonial empire that denied freedom to millions of people. Another duty is to examine anew the standard arguments that have been used to justify war; the argument that wars are fought out of necessity, in particular, raises the question of alternatives; this, Steinkraus maintains, has rarely been adequately investigated. The problem of human values is another one which needs scrutiny; modern war, he argues, violates all personal values, as does the very preparation for war.

Steinkraus is certainly right in wanting to redress the balance, since all too often philosophers have, as he demonstrates, fallen in with the rest of society in praising the virtues of war instead of exercising a moderating influence by not letting their emotions and passions prevail over reason and common sense. In the end we must, however, reflect upon the extraordinary range of individual human attitudes which contribute to the continued tolerance of war—which, in terms of the personal ends of the individual, is a demand that he convert the drive to preserve his own life into a drive to sacrifice it. As Julius Stone has commented, "merely rational motives of economic interest and the like are obviously ineffective to produce such alchemy; the deepest emotional convictions and the most firmly held ideals, however misguided, also obviously play their part. And the perplexities of men's age-old and ever-changing search for the good and the true and the holy are thus also close to the heart of the so-called 'problem of war.'"[87]

NOTES

1. Stanislav Andreski, "Pacifism and Human Nature," in Peter van den Dungen (ed.), *West European Pacifism and the Strategy for Peace* (London: Macmillan, 1985), 5.
2. Armand Clesse, "The Peace Movements and the Future of West European Security," in *ibid.*, 60.
3. Paul Vallely, "Walking the Warhead Road," *The Times,* July 11, 1986, 14. The fact that Kent refers to weapons, not war, is indicative of the evolution referred to. Kent's interlocutor continues: "Indeed, he feels as strongly about the perils of peaceful nuclear power. That, too, he sees as some kind of perversion of the natural order." One may well query both the reality of the existence, and the alleged beneficence, of "the natural order." Several practices which are now regarded as barbaric were once defended as belonging to that order. It is not long ago, either, that war itself was held to be a divine judgment and an integral part of that order.
4. See, e.g., David Henshaw, "Animal Liberationists Declare War on their own Species," *The Listener,* June 19, 1986, 4–5.
5. Karl Mannheim, *Man and Society in an Age of Reconstruction* (London: Kegan Paul, 1941), 41.
6. W.E.H. Lecky, *History of European Morals,* vol. 1 (London: Watts, 1930), 121.
7. *Ibid.,* 122.
8. *Ibid.*
9. *Ibid.* The observation that amusement, rather than learning about death, was Spinoza's intention seems to be borne out by the fact that in all his writings there is only one short sentence on death. Cf. Panos D. Bardis, *History of Thanatology: Philosophical, Religious, Psychological and Sociological Ideas Concerning Death from Primitive Times to the Present* (Washington, D.C.: University Press of America, 1981), 1 & 66. It is perhaps not surprising that in less than 100 pages, Bardis is unable to do justice to his subject: the title promises much more than the book delivers.
10. W.E.H. Lecky, *History, op. cit.,* 122.
11. W.E.H. Lecky, *History of European Morals,* vol. 2. (London: Watts, 1930), 8.
12. *Ibid.*
13. *Ibid.,* 10. He observes that the reforms of Christianity in this sphere were powerfully sustained by a doctrine "which is, perhaps, the most revolting in the whole theology of the Fathers." They taught that at the moment when the fetus in the womb acquired animation, it became an immortal being, which, in its unbaptized state, was doomed to be excluded forever from heaven. This doctrine is somewhat similar to the argument frequently used by early Quakers and some later non-Quaker pacifists that

it was better to be killed by an assailant than to kill him. The reasoning, in the words of Thomas Chalkley, an 18th-century English Quaker, being as follows: "That I being innocent, if I was killed in my body, my soul might be happy; but if I killed him, he dying in his wickedness, would consequently be unhappy; and if I was killed, he might live to repent; but if I killed him, he would have no time to repent; so that if he killed me, I should have much the better, both in respect to myself and to him." Cf. Peter Brock, *Pacifism in the United States* (Princeton: Princeton University Press, 1968), 79, note 102. After having quoted a similar view, Brock comments: "a curious argument, perhaps, to us today but one quite frequently urged by pacifist writers of the evangelical age."(492).

14. Although Christianity is one of the most pacifistic of faiths, Christian peoples have a record of military activity second to none. See, e.g., John Ferguson, *War and Peace in the World's Religions* (London: Sheldon Press, 1977), 122.

15. W.E.H. Lecky, *History, vol. 2, op. cit.,* 21.

16. *Ibid.*

17. Peter Brock, *Pacifism, op. cit.,* 52.

18. *Ibid.*

19. *Ibid.,* 94, note 37.

20. *Ibid.,* 504. Grimké was, however, opposed to capital punishment. When William Penn started his "Holy Experiment" in Pennsylvania in 1683, neither he nor his fellow Quakers held a testimony against capital punishment. It is only fair to point out that this penalty was retained, however, for only two offenses, murder and treason, at a time when in the mother country a multitude of offenses were punished by death.

21. The struggle between "compartmentation" and "inclusiveness"—and the resulting prevarication—as regards the agenda of the emerging peace movement can be followed, e.g., in the pages of *The Herald of Peace,* the organ of the London Peace Society. See, e.g., the editorial comment justifying the publication of an article entitled "On the Abolition of the Punishment of Death" in the April-June 1824 issue (89). Another essay on the same topic was published in the October–December issue (245).

22. George C. Beckwith in Thomas C. Upham, *The Manual of Peace* (Boston: American Peace Society, 1842), 7–8.

23. *Ibid.,* 100.

24. *Ibid.,* 152–153.

25. Peter Brock, *Pacifism, op. cit.,* 650.

26. George C. Beckwith, *The Peace Manual* (Boston: American Peace Society, 1847), Preface.

27. Peter Brock, *Pacifism, op. cit.,* 505.

28. *Ibid.,* 621–622.

29. *Ibid.*

30. *Ibid.*

31. *Ibid.*, 620.
32. John Sheppard, *An Inquiry on the Duty of Christians with Respect to War; Including an Examination of the Principles of the London and American Peace Societies* (London: T. Hamilton, 1820), 54–55, note. More recently, the same point has been made thus: "Strictly speaking...in spite of the fact that the term 'war' is applied to both aggressive activity and the activity of self-defense, an analysis of the respective activities will reveal that the two are contrary in most respects...if an instance of violence is a case of self-defense, then it is 'war' only in an incidental sense. Strictly, a 'war of self-defense' implies a contradiction in terms." Cf. A.C. Genova, "Can War be Rationally Justified?" in Robert Ginsberg (ed.), *The Critique of War: Contemporary Philosophical Explorations* (Chicago: Henry Regnery, 1969), 213.
33. Peter Brock, *Pacifism, op. cit.*, 699.
34. *Ibid.*, 696.
35. Ralph B. Potter, *War and Moral Discourse* (Richmond, Virginia: John Knox Press, 1969), 60. This is an excellent little volume with a substantial bibliographical essay (87–123).
36. *Ibid.*, 61.
37. *Ibid.*, 61–66.
38. D.B. Robertson (ed.), *Love and Justice: Selections from the Shorter Writings of Reinhold Niebuhr* (Cleveland, Ohio: World Publ. Comp./Meridian, 1967), 266–267. In another essay in the same collection, writing on pacifism and the use of force, Niebuhr comments: "The writer abhors consistency as a matter of general principle because history seems to prove that absolute consistency usually betrays into some kind of absurdity.(248) I fail to remember the author of the saying that consistency leads to the devil."
39. Peter Brock, *Pacifism, op. cit.*, 690–691.
40. *Ibid.*
41. John Lewis, *The Case against Pacifism* (London: George Allen & Unwin, 1940), 62.
42. *Ibid.*, 40.
43. It would be wrong to believe, however, that Franklin or Cicero were pacifists. Once Franklin had put the responsibility for the war of 1776 firmly on Great Britain, his denunciations of the war shifted from considerations of its inhumanity to those of its injustice, and peace as such ceased to be the ultimate goal of his actions. In 1778, e.g., he wrote: "Assure yourself, that nobody more sincerely wishes perpetual Peace among Men than I do; but there is a prior Wish, that they would be equitable and just, otherwise such Peace is not possible, and indeed wicked Men have no right to expect it." It was better to continue the War than "to submit to any base Conditions that may be offered us." Justice in international relations, then, might require the subordination of peace to its demands. See Gerald Stourzh, *Benjamin Franklin and American*

Foreign Policy, 2nd edition (Chicago: The University of Chicago Press, 1969), 186–190. Gerardo Zampaglione discusses Cicero's ideas on war and peace under the significant heading "Ciceronian Eclecticism": Cicero condemned war in the abstract but accepted and, indeed, extolled it in cases of legitimate defense, retaliation, or revenge. A more accurate expression of his view is that "the only excuse...for going to war is that we may live in peace unharmed." Cf. *The Idea of Peace in Antiquity* (Notre Dame: University of Notre Dame Press, 1973), 148–151.

44. John Oman, *The War and Its Issues*, quoted in Lewis, *Case, op. cit.*, 89.

45. Alan and Veronica Palmer, *Quotations in History* (Brighton: Harvester, 1976), 108.

46. John Lewis, *Case, op. cit.*, 30.

47. *Ibid.*, 78–84.

48. *Ibid.*, 85.

49. *Ibid.*, 123. In his cogently-argued book, Lewis takes issue with the views underlying a rational, secular pacifism. He argues, e.g., that violence does *not* always increase the sum of wickedness; that war does *not* always lead to more war; that one *can* extirpate evil with evil without becoming evil oneself. Only his chapters on the causes of war and on Russia reveal Lewis's Marxist bias. The attempt by Carl Marzani in his introduction to a modern reprint to stand the book on its head and use its arguments to make a case *for* pacifism is only partially successful. But Marzani is obviously right in asserting that "thermonuclear war strengthens the case for pacifism" since such a war would be self-defeating and "there isn't anything more evil than the extermination of the species." (New York: Garland, 1973), 9.

50. Louis J. Swift, "Augustine on War and Killing: Another View," *Harvard Theological Review* 66:3, July 1973, 375.

51. *Ibid.*, 377.

52. *Ibid.*, 382.

53. Arnold Toynbee, "Death in War," in Arnold Toynbee *et.al.*, *Man's Concern with Death* (London: Hodder and Stoughton, 1968), 146.

54. Sigmund Freud, "Thoughts for the Times on War and Death," (1915) in his *Civilization, War and Death*, John Rickman (ed.) (London: The Hogarth Press, 1939), 21.

55. *Ibid.*, 16–17.

56. *Ibid.*

57. J. Glenn Gray, *The Warriors: Reflections on Men in Battle* (New York: Harper and Row, 1967), 43.

58. *Ibid.*, 45.

59. *Ibid.*, 216.

60. *Ibid.*, 40.

61. *Ibid.*, XIV.

62. *Ibid.*, 46.

63. Cf. John Ferguson, *War and Peace, op. cit.,* 17.

64. Lecky has drawn the following analogy between the monastic and the military spirit: both "promote and glorify passive obedience, and therefore prepare the minds of men for despotic rule; but, on the whole, the monastic spirit is probably more hostile to freedom than the military spirit, for the obedience of the monk is based upon humility, while the obedience of the soldier co-exists with pride. Now, a considerable measure of pride, or self-assertion, is an invariable characteristic of free communities" (W.E.H. Lecky, *History, vol. 2, op. cit.,* 79). This seems, in a more general context, to be a case of standing Bernard Mandeville's fable on its head, since private virtues result in public vices. Earlier in his book, Lecky says as much when he observes: "Not infrequently...by a curious moral paradox, political crimes are closely connected with national virtues. A people who are submissive, gentle and loyal fall by reason of these very qualities under a despotic government."(*Ibid.,* vol.1, 64.) The moral ambiguity of obedience—a virtue which tends to become a vice—is well demonstrated in Stanley Milgram's classic study, *Obedience to Authority* (London: Tavistock, 1974). See also Alex Comfort, *Peace and Disobedience* (London: Peace News, 1946) and Francis Tuker, *The Pattern of War* (London: Cassell, 1948). Tuker quotes Robert G. Ingersoll's contention that history shows, again and again, that we have been saved by disobedience (and led to ruin by obedience). According to Sir Basil Liddell Hart, "We learn from history that the critics of authority have always been rebuked in self-righteous tones—if no worse fate has befallen them—yet have repeatedly been justified by history. To be 'agin the government' may be a more philosophic attitude than it appears." *Why Don't We Learn from History?* (London: George Allen & Unwin, 1944), 17. He goes on to relate this to the nature of governments which have an inherent tendency "to infringe the standards of decency and truth." Liddell Hart and others have shown that this adage applies with particular force to a country's defense establishment.

65. J. Glenn Gray, *Warriors, op. cit.,* 47–48.

66. *Ibid.,* 141–166.

67. *Ibid.,* 102.

68. Denis Winter, *Death's Men: Soldiers of the Great War* (Harmondsworth: Penguin Books, 1979), 181.

69. *Ibid.,* 181, 189, 210.

70. Hans J. Morgenthau, "Death in the Nuclear Age," *Politics in the Twentieth Century,* abbr. edition (Chicago: The University of Chicago Press, 1971), 202.

71. Richard A. Falk, *Law, Morality and War in the Contemporary World* (New York: Frederick A. Praeger, 1963), 45.

72. F.S. Northedge, "Peace, War, and Philosophy," in Paul Edwards (ed.), *The Encyclopedia of Philosophy,* vol. 6 (New York: Macmillan Comp. & The

Free Press, 1967), 66.

73. However, the "better red than dead" option, the belief that the values of freedom and liberty can be traded in for a war-free future existence is unlikely to be available: a more likely outcome of unilateral abandonment by the West of its military potential is a world of warring totalitarian powers in which many people will find themselves both "red and dead." See, e.g., Alexander Shtromas, "Pacifism and the Contemporary International Situation," in Peter van den Dungen (ed.), *West European Pacifism*, 34–50.

74. Paul Edwards (ed.), *Encyclopedia, op. cit.*, 66. Northedge's inaccurate presentation of Russell's views appears to be the result of a careless use of his sources.

75. Bertrand Russell, *Unpopular Essays* (London: George Allen and Unwin, 1970), 45.

76. Bertrand Russell, *Common Sense and Nuclear Warfare* (London: George Allen and Unwin, 1959), 90 (cf. appendix II, "Inconsistency?").

77. *Ibid.*, 88.

78. The view that it is always wrong for a government to start a war, and always right for it to meet external aggression with force, is simplistic. A preventive war against Nazi Germany in the 1930s might have been morally right, just as a defensive war in Czechoslovakia in 1968 might have been morally wrong (the latter because of the absence of a prospect of success.) Cf. Jonathan Glover, *Causing Death and Saving Lives* (Harmondsworth: Penguin Books, 1977), 269. The chapter "War," 251–285, is an excellent exposition of the moral issues involved.

79. Cf. Ralph Barton Perry, "What is Worth Fighting For?," *Atlantic Monthly* (December 1915), esp. 830, and reprinted in Charles Chatfield (ed.), *The Ethics of War: Bertrand Russell and Ralph Barton Perry on World War I*, (New York: Garland, 1972).

80. Bertrand Russell, "The Ethics of War," *International Journal of Ethics* (January 1915), 127–142, and contained in his *Justice in War-Time* (London: Open Court Publ., 1917), 19-37 (this volume is also reprinted in Charles Chatfield (ed.), *The Ethics of War, op. cit.*).

81. Ralph Barton Perry, "Non-Resistance and the Present War: A Reply to Mr. Russell," *International Journal of Ethics* (April 1915), 307–316, and reprinted in Charles Chatfield (ed.), *The Ethics of War, op. cit.* The quote is at 311.

82. *The Autobiography of Bertrand Russell, 1914–1944*, vol. II (London: George Allen and Unwin, 1968), 191.

83. *Ibid.*, 192.

84. Ralph Barton Perry, "Non-Resistance," *op. cit.*, 310; Bertrand Russell, "The War and Non-Resistance: A Rejoinder to Professor Perry," *International Journal of Ethics* (October 1915), 23–30, and reprinted in Charles Chatfield (ed.), *The Ethics of War, op. cit.* The quote is at 26.

85. H.G. Wells, *The War that will End War* (London: Frank and Cecil Palmer, 1914), 11.
86. Warren E. Steinkraus, "War and the Philosopher's Duty," in Robert Ginsberg (ed.), *Critique of War, op. cit.* 3–29.
87. Julius Stone, *Legal Controls of International Conflict* (New York: Rinehart, 1954), XXXV–XXXVI.

BIBLIOGRAPHY

Panos D. Bardis, *History of Thanatology: Philosophical, Religious, Psychological, and Sociological Ideas Concerning Death from Primitive Times to the Present* (Washington, D.C.: University Press of America, 1981).

George C. Beckwith, *The Peace Manual* (Boston: American Peace Society, 1847).

Peter Brock, *Pacifism in the United States* (Princeton University Press, 1968).

Charles Chatfield (ed.), *The Ethics of War: Bertrand Russell and Ralph Barton Perry on World War I* (New York: Garland, 1972).

Alex Comfort, *Peace and Disobedience* (London: Peace News, 1946).

Richard A. Falk, *Law, Morality and War in the Contemporary World* (New York: Frederick A. Praeger, 1963).

John Ferguson, *War and Peace in the World's Religions* (London: Sheldon Press, 1977).

Sigmund Freud, *Civilization, War and Death,* John Rickman (ed.) (London: The Hogarth Press, 1939).

Robert Ginsberg (ed.), *The Critique of War: Contemporary Philosophical Explorations* (Chicago: Henry Regnery, 1969).

Jonathan Glover, *Causing Death and Saving Lives* (Harmondsworth: Penguin Books, 1977).

J. Glenn Gray, *The Warriors: Reflections on Men in Battle* (New York: Harper and Row, 1967).

David Henshaw, "Animal Liberationists Declare War on their own Species," *The Listener,* June 19, 1986, 4–5.

W.E. H. Lecky, *History of European Morals* (London: Watts, 1930).

John Lewis, *The Case against Pacifism* (London: George Allen and Unwin, 1940).

Basil Liddell Hart, *Why Don't We Learn from History?* (London: George Allen and Unwin, 1944).

Karl Mannheim, *Man and Society in an Age of Reconstruction* (London: Kegan Paul, 1941).

Stanley Milgram, *Obedience to Authority* (London: Tavistock, 1974).

Hans J. Morgenthau, *Politics in the Twentieth Century* abr. edition (Chicago: The University of Chicago Press, 1971).

Reinhold Niebuhr, *Love and Justice: Selections from the Shorter Writings of Reinhold Niebuhr,* D.B. Robertson (ed.) (Cleveland, Ohio: World Publ. Co./Meridian, 1967).

F.S. Northedge, "Peace, War, and Philosophy" in Paul Edwards (ed.), *The Encyclopedia of Philosophy,* vol. 6 (New York: Macmillan Co. and The Free Press, 1967), 63–67.

Alan and Veronica Palmer, *Quotations in History* (Brighton: Harvester, 1976).

Ralph B. Potter, *War and Moral Discourse* (Richmond, Virginia: John Knox Press, 1969).

Bertrand Russell, *Justice in War-Time* (London: Open Court Publ., 1917).

Bertrand Russell, *Unpopular Essays* (London: George Allen and Unwin, 1970).

Bertrand Russell, *Common Sense and Nuclear Warfare* (London: George Allen and Unwin, 1959).

Bertrand Russell, *The Autobiography of Bertrand Russell, 1914–1944,* vol. II (London: George Allen and Unwin, 1968).

John Sheppard, *An Inquiry on the Duty of Christians with Respect to War; Including an Examination of the Principles of the London and American Peace Societies* (London: T. Hamilton, 1820).

Julius Stone, *Legal Controls of International Conflict* (New York: Rinehart, 1954).

Gerald Stourzh, *Benjamin Franklin and American Foreign Policy* 2nd edition (Chicago: The University of Chicago Press, 1969).

Louis J. Swift, "Augustine on War and Killing: Another View," *Harvard Theological Review* 66:3 (July 1973), 369–383.

Arnold Toynbee, *et. al.*, *Man's Concern with Death* (London: Hodder and Stoughton, 1968).

Francis Tuker, *The Pattern of War* (London: Cassell, 1948).

Thomas C. Upham, *The Manual of Peace* (Boston: American Peace Society, 1842).

Paul Vallely, "Walking the Warhead," *The Times*, July 11, 1986, 4.

Peter van den Dungen (ed.) *West European Pacifism and the Strategy for Peace* (London: Macmillan, 1985).

H.G. Wells, *The War that will End War* (London: Frank and Cecil Palmer, 1914).

Denis Winter, *Death's Men: Soldiers of the Great War* (Harmondsworth: Penguin Books, 1979).

Gerardo Zampaglione, *The Idea of Peace in Antiquity* (Notre Dame: University of Notre Dame Press, 1973).

CONTRIBUTORS

Paul Badham Professor of Theology and Religious Studies and Dean of the Faculty of Theology, St. David's University, Lampeter, University of Wales.

Michael Coughlan Dean of Faculty of Arts and Senior Lecturer in Philosophy, St. David's University College, Lampeter, University of Wales.

Christie Davies Professor of Sociology, University of Reading, England.

Simon Fishel Scientific Director, Human In-vitro Fertilization Unit, The Park Hospital, and Senior Lecturer in Obstetrics and Gynecology, University of Nottingham, England.

Nicholas Kittrie Professor of Law and Director of the Institute of Law and Policy, American University, Washington D.C., USA.

Shigemi Kono Director General, Institute of Population Problems, Ministry of Health and Welfare, Tokyo, Japan.

Jan Kryspin Assistant Professor of Physiology and Rehabilitation Medicine, University of Toronto, Canada.

Helga Kuhse Deputy Director and Research Fellow, Center for Human Bioethics, Monash, Australia.

Heather Phillips Research Fellow in Medieval Studies, University of Toronto, Canada.

Peter Singer Professor of Philosophy and Director of the Center for Human Bioethics, Monash, Australia.

Patrick Nowell Smith Emeritus Professor of Philosophy, York University, Ontario, Canada.

Peter van den Dungen Lecturer in Peace Studies, University of Bradford, England.

Robert Winston Director of In-vitro Fertilization Program, Hammersmith Hospital, and Professor of Obstetrics and Gynecology, University of London, England.

SOURCES

The content of this volume was derived from papers presented in Committee II ("The Value of Human Life") at ICUS XV ("Absolute Values and the New Cultural Revolution"). The symposium, one of seven sponsored by ICUS, was held at the J.W. Marriott Hotel in Washington, D.C., November 27–30, 1986, and was chaired by Honorary Chairman Claude A. Villee, Jr. and Organizing Chairman Paul Badham.

Index

CHAPTER 9 (continued)
page 204, note 9, line 3;
. . .Sixth World Congress on Care of the. . .
page 205, note 17, line 3;
. . .Current Crisis in Medicine - a Plea for a Philosophical. . .
page 206, note 34, line 1;
. . .Brief, sensitive treatments of the question. . .

CHAPTER 10
page 215, quote indent, last line;
. . .once wrote, "not only those of nature's cruelty or doctors' ingenuity.". .

CHAPTER 11
page 223, line 6;
. . .glory of their masters.". . .
page 224, paragraph 2, line 8;
. . .critic of the current peace movement to write of its members. . .
page 225, line 9;
. . .literally, declared war on vivisectors.. . .
page 228, quote indent, line 3;
. . .inter-national war and has nothing to do with anything. . .
page 229, paragraph 2, line 5;
. . .only the admissibility of defensive war. . .
page 231, 2nd quote indent, line 3;
. . .ideas; because it includes *contrary things*,. . .
page 232, paragraph 1, line 18;
. . .vigorously supported prosecution of the war. . .
page 234, paragraph 2, line 3;
. . .has been spilled lightly and immorally,. . .
page 235, line 4 from page bottom;
. . .denied by pacifists, namely that between killing and murder. . .
page 238, paragraph 2, line 21;
. . .reasons for fighting, such reasons being to. . .
page 242, line 20 and 21;
. . .utter defeat. I found this possibility unbearable, and at last consciously
and definitely decided that. . .
— — line 10 from page bottom;
. . .hated war, and to Perry's claim that "the one cause for. . .
page 246, note 38 line 6 and 7;
. . .consistency usually betrays into some kind of absurdity." (248) I fail to
remember the author of the saying that consistency leads to the devil.. . .
page 252, line 8;
Paul Vallely, "Walking the Warhead Road" *The Times*, July 11, 1986, 4.. . .

CHAPTER 9
page 181, line 5;
. . .a state of chronic dis-ease,. . .
− − paragraph 3, line 3;
. . .resulted, in the last 20 years,. . .
page 182, paragraph 1, line 4 and 5;
. . .principles are applied to the care of the terminally ill has been
demonstrated by Dr. Edmund Pellegrino,. . .
page 183, last three lines;
. . .progressive devaluation of life, as witnessed by the recent history of
court decisions in the US - Quinlan (1976), Conroy (1983 - 1984),. . .
page 184, paragraph 1, line 14;
. . .compassion and the affective and spiritual support due. . .
page 187, paragraph 1, line 2;
. . .are proposing here goes against current moral trends. . .
page 188, last two lines;
. . .things cannot be achieved without cost. "If doctors could learn,"
Katz argues,. . .
page 190, last four lines,
  Here, drawing briefly on the work of some of the most skilled clinicians
(those who have attempted to be fully present to the dying patient and to
share that reality) we shall indicate what are most commonly. . .
page 192, paragraph 1, line 1 and 2
  Having perceived some of the needs of the dying person, we now ask
what can be done. . .
− − paragraph 3, last three lines;
. . .management. Our purpose here is simply to suggest a new and. . .
page 195, paragraph 2, line 4;
. . .ill patient. The issue of confidentiality has been addressed by Margaret
Somerville.. . .
page 197 paragraph 2, line 1;
Refusal of Treatment. When treatment is refused,. . .
− − line 11;
. . .accept medical treatment, even if refusal may result in. . .
page 201, line 14;
. . .act as a catalyst to growth (if simply to assist. . .
− − line 17 and 18;
. . .Furthermore, if the doctor-patient relationship is truly genuine, the
patient will act as a catalyst in the doctor's. . .
page 203, paragraph 2, heading;
Summary
page 204, note 5;
. . .P. Laslett, *The World We Have Lost*, 103-04.. . .
− − note 6, line 2;
. . .Stanford University Press, 1958) 236-237.. . .

CHAPTER 6 (continued)

page 111, line 4;

. . .(The state's right to execute did, however, live on. . .

— — paragraph 1, line 9;

. . .overriding importance of these values by taking. . .

— — paragraph 3, line 10;

. . .the sections of the American Law Institute's Model Penal Code. . .

page 112, paragraph 3, line 1 and 2;

The abolitionists, knowing they were winning the causalist arguments, were apparently willing. . .

page 125, line 3, new sentences;

. . .It may take a very long time. At present the number of individuals being executed is still low by the standards of the past, however it is rising and is likely to continue to rise during the 1990s.. . .

page 130, note 3;

. . .and Amnesty International 1989, 1990, 1991.. . .

page 133, SELECT BIBLIOGRAPHY, new entries after first reference;

- Amnesty International, When the State Kills, London, Amnesty International, 1989.. . .

- Amnesty International, Amnesty International (Annual) Report London, Amnesty International, 1990.. . .

- Amnesty International, USA: *The Death Penalty in the United States of America: Developments from 1 September, 1989 to 31 December, 1990,* London, Amnesty International, 1991.. . .

page 135, Selected American Supreme Court Cases, line 7;

       Harris v. McRae (1980). . .

CHAPTER 8

page 156, last line;

. . .theoretical issues issues for later.. . .

page 157, paragraph 1, lines 4, 5 and 6;

. . .States of America in 1982, following the death of "Baby Doe.". . .

page 175, paragraph 1, line 6;

. . .make informed decisions if they are carefully and. . .

— — paragraph 3, line 1 and 2;

Many people draw a moral distinction between doing or omitting to do something that results in death,. . .

page 176, ACKNOWLEDGEMENTS, line 1;

Parts of this article are drawn from a book jointly authored by Helga Kuhse and Peter Singer: *Should the Baby Live?,*...

— — line 3;

. . .drawn from a joint article. . .

ERRATA
ETHICS ON THE FRONTIERS
OF HUMAN EXISTENCE
Edited by Paul Badham

CHAPTER 2
page 46, paragraph 2, line 5;
...embryo research, the 20,000 healthy babies already...
— — paragraph 3, line 2;
...In the U.K. so far, less than 7,000 babies have...
— — paragraph 3, line 5;
...needed. IVF remains one of the least successful...
page 47, line 1;
...Paradoxically, it is still relatively unsuccessful....
— — paragraph 2, line 4 and 5;
...Ectopic pregnancy can cause massive abdominal hemorrhage and
sufferers often require...
page 48, paragraph 1, line 11;
...or lead hopelessly inhuman lives,...
— — paragraph 2, line 4;
...fetus is deformed. Yet, the British Parliament until recently showed
great hesitation...

CHAPTER 4
page 70, line 1;
...endorsed the "Pauline principle" (page 66, above),...
page 71, paragraph 1, line 7;
...is taken to be something good.....
page 77, paragraph 1, line 18;
...What, e.g., has been done by the obstetrician who...
page 79, note 3, line 2;
...Society, 1968), (hereafter *Humanae Vitae*) $14.

CHAPTER 6
page 102, paragraph 1, line 8, new sentence;
...Within the last decade the falling trend has been reversed but so far
the actual number of executions is much lower than it was before 1965.
— — Table 6-1, line 7, new lines 8 and 9;
1970-79 - - - 03
1980-84 - - - 29
1985-89 - - - 88
page 105, next to last line;
...and religious issues were played down and controversial...